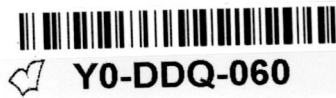

THE

Healer's

Call

CHRIST-CENTERED
ENERGY HEALERS
and THEIR STORIES

Book Two

THE
Healer's
Call

CHRIST-CENTERED
ENERGY HEALERS
and THEIR STORIES

Book Two

Inner Light Press
a Silver Torch Press company

The Healer's Call: Book Two
Christ-Centered Energy Healers & Their Stories

Copyright © 2016 by Hope Haven Events

Published by Inner Light Press, an imprint of Silver Torch Press
www.SilverTorchPress.com
Jill@SilverTorchPress.com

ISBN 978-1-942707-24-0

Book design by KayLynn Flanders
Compiled by Tammy Ward
Edited by Jamie Garlick

Contents

PREFACE

This book is a compilation book full of stories on how these amazing men and women came to know energy healing that is Christ-centered to them. Hope Haven Events makes no claims on what others will experience. However, we have been invited by our Heavenly Father to collect and share some of these incredible stories of healing and how these experiences have brought them closer to their Savior. You may not be able to relate to all of them, but chances are you will be able to connect to some of them.

At Hope Haven Events, our mission is to empower individuals, strengthen families and connect communities. We are grateful for the thousands who have attended our conferences and events, read our books, listened to our audios, and participated in our mentoring and other online programs. We value you greatly.

Much love,

Tammy Anderson Ward
& the whole team at Hope Haven Events

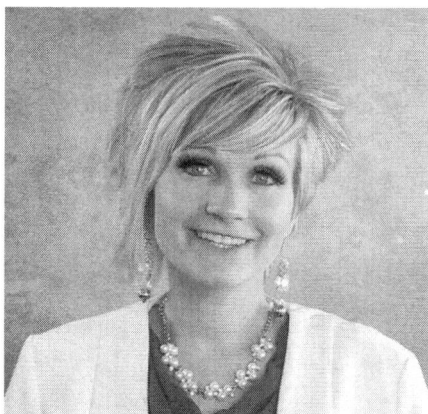

TAMMY WARD

Tammy Ward is the President of Hope Haven Events. They host several conferences including the Christ-centered Energy Healing Conference, Winter Homeschool Conference and more, retreats, online group mentoring experiences and specialty events to help accomplish Tammy's passion of "empowering individuals, strengthening families and connecting communities."

Along with her own events, Tammy also actively speaks professionally worldwide. She is responsible for this compilation book series, The Healer's Call & The Holistic Ways Journal. She loves working on fun projects & helping others to feel better.

Tammy is also a homeschooling mom to 8 awesome kids. She is best known for being a fun and inspirational mover and shaker! She has learned a great deal from her real life experiences with holistic health, miracles, and in overcoming addictions by trusting Heavenly Father and her Savior, Jesus Christ. She is certified in many energy healing modalities simply because she loves to make others feel better and heal naturally.

She is grateful for the many healing blessings she has experienced. These are just a few of the stories that her family has been so grateful for.

"A Burning Desire To Be Healed"

I had been in the kitchen cooking my family dinner, when all of the sudden my six year old little boy started screaming with a desperate, painful cry. He quickly joined me as he ran from the family room straight away into the kitchen. His entire back was engulfed in flames.

The back of his hair was literally on fire and I began to quickly panic. I attempted to extinguish the flames by smothering them with my fingertips in a quick, patting motion. I realized that I was actually fanning those flames, making them grow. It was a pretty intense moment, and I had to decide on something more efficient very quickly or this was going to get worse.

I pulled off his shirt from the bottom up and threw it on the tiled, kitchen floor. I then grabbed his hand and took him quickly into the bathroom. I was about ready to put him under the shower with cold, water running on his back when all of the sudden an urgent voice inside me said, "No. Stop."

An image appeared in my mind of a salve that I had bought two weeks previous to this incident. We laid him down and I quickly went for it. He was screaming in agony at first as I carefully spread it quite thick onto his back.

You may be wondering why I hadn't just taken him to the hospital as this was an emergency. I mean, I fully recognize that a person would normally take their son to the hospital for such an emergency. However, I waited to see what God wanted me to do. I asked Him if I should go to the hospital. I believed that He would tell me the best option. He told me through the still, small voice that I should wait and to put some salve on his back, which I quickly did. I began to blow air out of my mouth onto my son's back, which offered him relief to the pain. Still to this day he remembers how good that helped it to feel.

Thirty minutes passed, and I felt like I was beginning to hyperventilate. I began to realize I was not going to be able to continue doing this for long. I could see the severity of this burn and knew he was a little boy. I was struggling inside of myself with what to do next.

I said a silent prayer to my Father in Heaven pleading for His assistance. Immediately after saying "amen" in my mind, I knew what to do. I called Courtney, my mentor who had been training me how to use energy medicine in my everyday life as well as for clients. She lived many hours away from me, but I wasn't worried. I knew about remote healing, which means the practitioner could do work on the person from a distance, using proxy. She is a very busy woman, so I was extremely grateful when she answered the phone. She had been a registered nurse and understands the anatomy and functions of the body better than almost anyone I know.

He quit crying within seconds. Then, he commented that he was cold. Courtney was giggling on the phone, and I couldn't understand why. Upon inquiring with her, she shared with me that she had just pulled the heat out of his back using energy medicine, of course. He didn't feel any pain after that point. Quickly the area on the small of his back where the skin and tissue had been melted began to change colors. Right before our eyes, we observed pink, healthy tissue emerging. We were so grateful. The entire wound healed quickly. We continued to apply the miracle salve. As an added measure, we also laid plastic wrap over the top to keep it clean and prevent it from drying out. Only a few times a day did we take that off and let it breathe.

If you look at my son's back, there is hardly a scar. He will tell you he knows energy medicine is legit. His burn injury healed so quickly that my friends and family were amazed. It made big believers out of many who weren't convinced of the legitimacy of what I was learning through the courses I was taking.

"How do I know muscle testing is okay with Heavenly Father?"

First of all, I take A LOT of precautions to make sure I am using His light. I have had personal revelation about this specifically and several sacred experiences. Pray about it, and do what feels best for you. Here is what I do:

- Before beginning, I ask in prayer for protection. You can do this by shielding, asking Heavenly Father to send angels to protect you or by simply asking for protection.
- I only ask questions that are specific, not general.
- I ask if I have Heavenly Father's permission. I literally say, "Do I have permission to test on this?"
- I double check if there is any question in my mind or heart at all. I do this by asking, "Am I using the LIGHT of CHRIST?" Another way to ask this is, "IS THIS TRUTH?" You can also ask the question, "Am I getting interference?"

I had a special experience this past week where it was revealed to me that it was not only okay, but it was what Heavenly Father wanted me to do.

From my Journal on May 24, 2014

"My family was preparing to go on a Family Trek with many other homeschool families. There were about 125 of us in all. I am in the very early stages of my pregnancy so with morning sickness, I wasn't super ecstatic about going, but I did want to be there for my family.

My husband, Casey had a general anesthesia surgery removing two of his wisdom teeth. When he was waking up in the recovery room, my son Kaden that was with us passed out when they were taking out the I.V. He has a weak stomach like his daddy, I guess. We had to wait for an additional hour because he was vomiting and having a rough time once he came to. <<< Actually, since then we have learned what an empath this kid really is. I am grateful to have learned shielding and other forms of Christ-centered protection. >>>

With all of this going on, I wasn't quite sure if we were supposed to go or not, but after getting the confirmation from Heavenly Father we knew we were supposed to go.

Like anytime I leave to go out of town now, I went over to my essential oils, herbs and tinctures, and asked with muscle testing what I should take with me. I have a simple prayer in my heart that my needs and the needs of my family will be taken care of while we are away from home. I ask if I have Heavenly Father's permission too. I usually don't take that much with me, but I am grateful for muscle testing (kinesiology) that I can figure out what to take.

The Trek

We had a very spiritual, bonding, uplifting experience as a family. Even though my feet blistered and I struggled physically, I grew spiritually while there. I could feel the gratitude of my ancestors. Interesting to think that they have gratitude for us, but there it was. I knew that they did. They are grateful they were being remembered for their faith. They are grateful we were honoring their sacrifice. They love us. They know us. They are more a part of us than we will ever understand. My testimony increased greatly.

I took a small case of essential oils and a couple other things with me. It was pretty neat to reflect on the fact that I ended up using the things I took with me and what we used them for.

- Lavender: Sunburns, scratches,
- Peppermint: Morning sickness/ nausea, cooling body temp down.

- MyGraine: Headaches.
- Orange Sweet: Uplifting, happy smell
- Cinnamon Bark: I put this on my wrists as we walked. I licked my wrists every now and again. It tasted like I had a mouth full of red hots. I know there are some other things that it probably helped with too.
- Serenity: We used at night to help us sleep.
- On Guard: As an infection prevention for my husband's mouth.
- Basil: A 12 year old girl in a camp next to ours ended up with an ear infection. This helped her greatly. She only needed to use it once and it was gone.
- Therma Care: A friend of mine that went ended up with dehydration and exhaustion. She walked over to me and told me she was dizzy. I had her sit down and took off her shoes. I rubbed her feet and used the Therma Care with her. I also had a mini bottle of concentrated minerals. I put some of that in her water too. I know it helped her.
- Energy: I sure used this one a lot. This is a blend made by Butterfly Express.
- Frankincense: A little girl got slammed into by a hand cart right in her hip. It sure helped her a lot.
- BBL: This is a natural pain reliever that is a tincture from Butterfly Express also. This helped several people.
- Arnica: We used this great homeopathy for not just my husband's mouth, but we also used it for our sore and tired muscles. IT WAS A HUGE HELP!!!
- Energy Work: WHOA. Love this. Thank you Heavenly Father for this knowledge. It has helped so many around me already.

I am so grateful that I have learned all of the tools and education. It has helped me to serve in a greater capacity, for sure. I love my

Heavenly Father so much and am so grateful that He has given us what we need. Muscle testing is not to replace prayer. Instead, it has brought me closer to my Savior and my Heavenly Father.

Placing One Foot In Front Of The Other...

There are many ways to put your body into complete homeostasis. If you are wondering about alternative health for your own family either to become self-reliant or in times of emergency preparedness, I would like to share with you the benefits of getting a mentor. A mentor is someone who can answer your questions and be a leader or a guide for you. Choose someone you trust. Be sure to choose someone who has a good relationship with Jesus Christ. Since getting a mentor last year, my family has been greatly blessed. We have agreed that we will always have a mentor from here on out. If you'd like to learn more about the mentoring that is offered directly through Hope Haven Events in regards to energy healing in a Christ-centered way, go to our website at energyhealingconference.com. You will also find audio recordings on all of our previous conferences. In addition, you can pick up our other books, programs, and even mentor with us there.

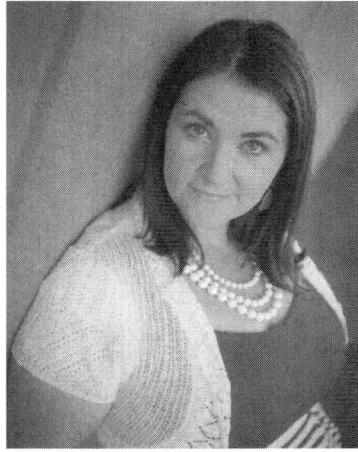

MINDY POWELL

Mindy Powell, Founder of Warrior Optimist, is a dynamic speaker, captivating writer, inspiring mentor, and energy healer. She has been featured in Women's World Magazine and GreenSmoothieGirl.com for her incredible journey to health and releasing over 100 lbs. Mindy has overcome many hard life experiences which enable her to provide understanding and influence the lives of many. She is passionate about empowering others to build their foundation on Christ, love themselves fiercely, and move forward with faith. Mindy candidly shares personal, engaging stories from her own beautiful, messy journey to inspire others to Choose Hope, Practice Courage, and Bloom Radiance.

Warrior Optimist

Choose Hope, Practice Courage, Bloom Radiance

I will never forget the day I came home and realized my life was falling apart. My heart was pounding out of control and I couldn't breathe. I was suffocating. I was drowning. I felt like I was in an awful abyss, a never-ending nightmare, and there was no way out. I wanted to give up. I wanted to be done with life. I couldn't see any purpose and felt no passion in anything. I was overwhelmed, stressed, hurt, crushed, beaten down, stuck, and pained deeply to my core. I had zero hope for the future. I wanted to lay down and die, but I didn't. I am so glad I somehow kept going.

I felt overwhelmed, complete and utter chaos, and confusion. Christ had always been important to me and a big part of my life. My proximity to the Savior had always been there, but I didn't naturally immerse myself completely in Him with all my body, mind and spirit. I was not always dependent on His presence.

I didn't truly feel His divine help in every aspect of my life as intensely as I desired. When my life continued to fall apart at the seams, it was then that I truly chose to become closer to Christ. I wanted to experience the power of healing through Christ, although I don't think I even knew exactly what that truly meant or what it felt like.

I yearned for truth and was seeking Christ's light in my life with all my heart. I desired to intimately know my Savior. I craved having complete faith and trust in Him to direct me in my life. I wanted to feel inspired and have my heart tell me the things that my conscious mind did not know.

I needed to feel divine revelation flowing freely through my soul. I wanted an unshakable trust in my Savior. I sought to have my life aligned with God's plan for me. I wanted to know what I truly believed in and why? I wanted to feel my purpose, know my gifts and feel passionate inside. I wanted to know me! I had lost myself through the years. I was ready to love myself and find me!

Everything in life was so intense and I continued to have one loss after another in my life. Whenever I thought I couldn't lose any more, I somehow did. It started with instability in my marriage. My husband was unfaithful and this caused me to feel tremendous hurt and

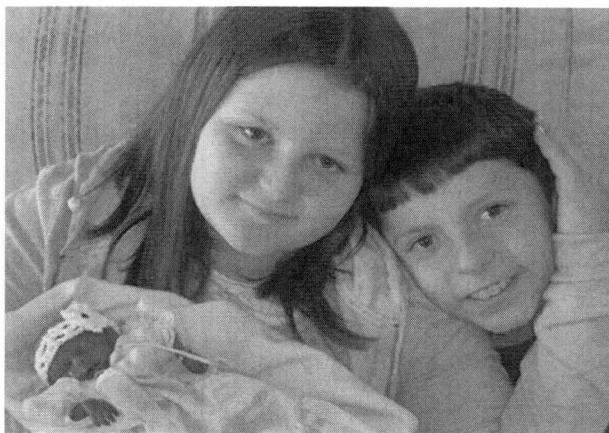

insurmountable heartache. I turned to Christ and fought hard for my marriage, but it was not to be. I found out I was pregnant just before my divorce was final. I suffered a debilitating pregnancy, alone and on bed rest.

After an emergency C-section, my baby lived only three days and I lost my baby as well.

I had lost my physical health, financial stability, my best friend of 20 years, and my sweet baby. It was all too much. I tail-spinned into deep depression and experienced severe suicidal thoughts. I felt like I had lost everything. I had nothing to live for.

I felt so *alone*! I wanted to *die* and I didn't think I would ever come back from these horrible *traumas*. I couldn't comprehend that any-one could hurt like me or had experienced this much pain. I felt like I was broken.

Everything was just too overwhelming in my life. Life was too hard. I was drowning fast in life and didn't know how to cope with the utter exhaustion. I felt so numb. I had no idea how my life had gotten to this point. All these yucky words were floating through my mind and taking over my inner being. Most of the time, I felt like all I was doing is simply surviving one more day of grief and pain. I somehow found the strength, hope and courage to persevere. I didn't realize at the time, but I had a small ray of hope still left inside of me. But most days, it was a struggle to even get out of bed and get dressed. During these hard struggles, I learned to wholeheartedly turn to Christ. I found hope and healing through Him. I have tremendous gratitude for everything I went through. I learned and progressed more than any other time in my life. I increased my personal relationship with my Savior Jesus Christ and Heavenly Father exponentially—more than the rest of my life combined. I wouldn't change any of my experiences. There are no accidents. There is great purpose and many reasons for everything that I went through.

I know one of the biggest reasons I made it through all of this trauma alive is because I kept trusting, building my foundation on Christ and allowing Him to heal me. I have vivid memories sitting in my chair in my bedroom focusing on several pictures of Christ and pouring through the scriptures, until I felt some sort of peace inside my tumultuous body.

I dug deep to find the strength and power within me to move forward. It was always there, I just had to discover it. I decided to love myself enough to take this journey; to find my true divinity and treasures inside of myself. I realized this power had always been within me; it was up to me to shape it, form it and let it shine through. I allowed this new power to pour through me like nothing I had ever experienced before. I immersed myself in Christ.

Growing up, I had been taught to have faith in Christ and was introduced to the concept of energy healing with things such as Reiki, essential oils and kinesiology, but nothing was done on a consistent basis. It was in the midst of my worst struggles in life when I truly discovered Christ-centered energy healing and became more acquainted with its profound impact on my life. I saw the results it had on my own healing.

I accepted Christ to carry my burdens. I allowed Him to make more of my life than I could possibly create on my own. I experienced so many tender mercies and miracles in my life. I discovered through the healing process that I could feel divine guidance flowing freely. I continued down my pathway of healing and found many tools to aid me on this journey.

I came to realize the profound importance of personal prayer every morning and night. I loved communing with God and pouring my heart and soul out to Him. I began to truly communicate with God on a more intimate level. I prayed like I had never prayed before. Instead of a quick two minute prayer in the morning, I found myself praying for sometimes hours at a time. I came to know the meaning of "pray always." I would often kneel in my closet and let my thoughts and feelings flow freely.

I remember one day my legs were aching so badly. I knew I hadn't done any exercise or strenuous activity. I

> "Trust in the Lord with all thine heart; and lean not unto thine own understanding. In all thy ways acknowledge him, and he shall direct thy paths." Proverbs 3:5-6

was stumped by the pain. The following day it hit me; my legs were hurting because I had been constantly on my knees in prayer. I wanted answers so deeply, I was willing to do whatever it took. I recognized the impact of feasting on the scriptures and taking time for myself to ponder things in my heart. I started to focus on Christ. I received powerful guidance and revelation through the scriptures and words of God.

I built my foundation on Christ in an intense way that I had never done before. Every morning, I studied the scriptures for direction in my life. This forever impacted me for good. Even at my hardest, darkest moments during my journey, I would read at least one scripture a day with my children. There were times when I didn't eat or sleep or when I wasn't even present. But I kept focusing on Christ, saying my prayers and reading scriptures.

I continued to find tools to add to my healing. I started processing and releasing negative emotions and energy that had been pent up inside. I realized I needed to release the negative and also fill myself up with positive beliefs and emotions.

Through following the Spirit, I was able to participate in a class on energy healing. This energy work was Christ-centered and gave me tremendous hope during my healing progression. I started looking within and developing my own spiritual gifts that had been hiding for so long. I also found great support through my new network of energy healing friends.

I had some powerful experiences with energy work. These instances are very sacred and spiritual. They had an intense impact on my healing and moving forward in life. One friend in my energy healing class was able to help me cut many negative connecting cords in my life that I had been struggling with for quite a while. It was a huge accomplishment!

"O Lord, give us strength according to our faith which is in Christ, even unto deliverance. And they broke the cords with which they were bound." –Alma 14:26

Another friend helped me see heart walls I had put up and how broken my heart was. She aided me in starting the process to protect and heal my heart. I learned so much about myself as I continued on my journey to heal. I realized how much we need one another. We are here on earth to help each other get back home. We can't do it alone. We need Christ and one another to help us.

"WE 'RE ALL JUST WALKING EACH OTHER HOME."

-Ram Dass

Mine was not an easy path of healing, but it was the perfect path for me. There were many months I felt like I was simply surviving in life. It felt like I was moving forward one step, and then backwards a hundred. I often felt very stuck in life and too overwhelmed to try.

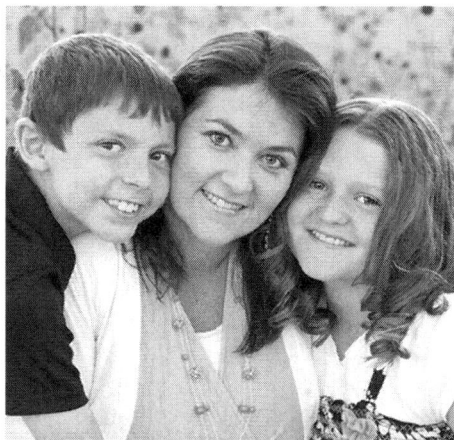

I prayed intently to be carried through my trials. I continually asked my heavenly guardians for help and support. I persisted in building my foundation on Christ. I constantly focused on Christ and allowed Him to help heal the intense suffering that had taken place in my life. I finally felt a small glimmer of hope!

Divine revelation started to *flow* inside of me. The Spirit exuded from my being and gave me *strength* and *direction* in life. I was constantly feeling inspired. I found my purpose and passion in life. I enjoyed being a loving mother again to my other two children.

I was focusing on amazing, powerful thoughts to create my new destiny! It was an absolutely incredible feeling inside of my body! I felt alive and radiant! I knew that with a sincere heart, real intent, and faith in Christ; I could have truth manifested to me through the Spirit. I knew Christ would tell me in my mind and in my heart what my next step was. I knew the Spirit was inside of me like a gift waiting to be opened. It was my choice to receive inspiration. It required effort and continual striving of knowledge on a daily basis. I had to do my part, but I also reaped the rewards.

I felt the power and peace inside of me as I linked with Christ and connected to Him in my life. I looked to Heaven for guidance in everything I did. My quality of life grew. The depth of joy I felt was utterly amazing. I felt clarity and direction in my life. I was devoted to finding truth and not settling for anything less.

My personal discernment increased. I could access spiritual strength whenever I sought after it. I desired everyone to feel this powerful spirit and direction in life. It became my life mission to help others feel the true happiness I felt. I wanted others to learn to utilize this amazing inspiration in life!

I love sharing my story to help inspire others on their own journey of hope and healing. I can truly testify with authenticity to all of my challenges. I have grown in ways I never would have been able to under any other circumstances. I have the ability to help many people and impact others for good.

I am constantly looking within myself and finding the power of Christ within me. I know that through Christ, I have everything inside of me to heal and move forward in faith and confidence in the future.

I believe we can heal all of our pain through Christ. We can place all our hurts in His hands and find healing through Christ.

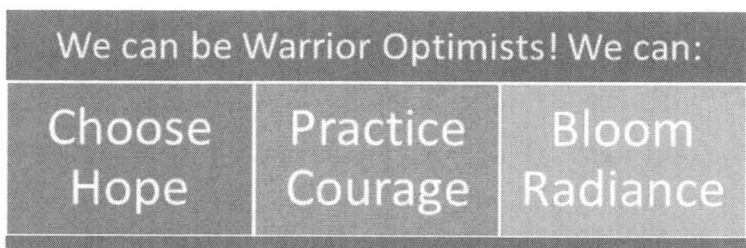

We can be Warrior Optimists! We can:		
Choose Hope	Practice Courage	Bloom Radiance

I would love to connect with you!
Mindy Powell
WarriorOptimist.com
WarriorOptimist@gmail.com

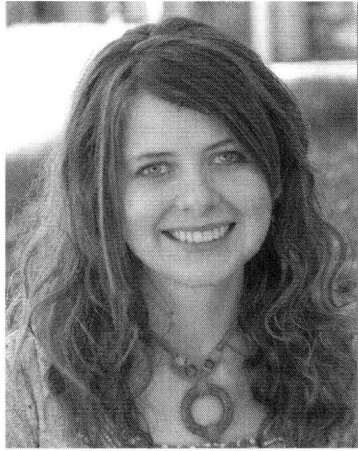

CASSIE HUGHES

Cassie Hughes is certified in the Emotion Code and Body Code modalities. She is currently certifying in three-dimensional therapy and is proficient in energy psychology. She spent a year training directly under Dr. Bradley Nelson and his staff, focusing her studies on relationship dynamics and inner-child work. Cassie works with clients who suffer from all kinds of physical and emotional problems from fibromyalgia to hormone imbalances and anger management to depression and anxiety. Cassie also enjoys being a mother, piano player and artist. For more information about Cassie's sessions, visit www.cassielhughes.com.

I grew up, like most of us, on pure western culture. I felt I had a happy childhood with a mom and dad who cared about me and an older brother who teased me relentlessly, just like it should be. I was a child full of wonder and imagination, and I had a free spirit that just wanted to play. In my mind, life was exciting and full of limitless possibilities; I could be anything.

The rest of my family, however, didn't see as much sunshine at home as I did. They are all very strong dominate types. My dad and brother were always fighting, while my mother suppressed her dominating personality in order to keep peace. This ended up causing quite a bit of unmentionable trauma in my parent's relationship. One day my parents told me they were getting divorced. I went to my room and just bawled, feeling my first heartbreak. I thought that maybe, if I cried hard enough, they wouldn't break up. My feelings were validated when they came in a couple hours later to tell me they were staying together and that they loved each other. It worked. In my mind, it was my tears that kept them together. After that moment, I always felt a sense of responsibility toward my family. It was up to me to keep them happy and together...a tall order for someone so small!

In a way, I was right. My mother decided to stay with my father initially because she didn't want to hurt her children. But the reasons why she wanted a divorce in the first place didn't get resolved. She buried her feelings so deeply, put on a straight face and kept living life to the best of her capability, for her children. That is when her health started rapidly declining. It started with debilitating migraines that became more and more frequent. These spiraled into more severe health problems. Over the next 20 years she was diagnosed with a myriad of diseases. Fibromyalgia, diabetes, arthritis, TMJ, Liver disease, depression, the list goes on. She went to many specialists and doctors, and ended up taking 20 pills a day at some points, but to no avail...she just kept getting sicker and sicker until she was in her bed, too weak to move, all day and all night.

At times, I wondered if her sickness had to do with emotional problems. But back then, that kind of notion was like saying, "Buck up, Mom, it's all in your head." And saying something like that would back-fire very quickly. So we kept trucking along in life the best we could manage, with my mother getting sicker and without any concrete answers. She ended up missing out on so much of life. She tried really hard to make it to the important things like recitals, concerts and graduations, but many times, she just couldn't. Rumors and lies about drug addictions and other problems started to circulate around in the community and church about her and why she was in bed all of the time. This made it extremely difficult for her to go to church or other social events, even if she did feel somewhat up for it. She always had a smile for me and never complained about her plight, at least not to me, but you could tell there was a deep sadness in her eyes, that life was not what she wanted it to be.

One day while driving to school, I let my emotions get the better of me and started focusing hopelessly on my mom's health. I questioned if she would ever get better. From time to time I would pray earnestly that she would heal, counting on my faith to get her there. She never did heal overnight like I expected, and that made me wonder if I didn't have enough faith. I felt that maybe it was me keeping her sick. As I was pondering these things, I drove my car up a big bend in the road on a hill and at the top of the hill was the most vibrant double rainbow I had ever seen. I was washed over with this incredible feeling that one rainbow represented my mother and the other represented me. My mother would heal in time, and even though I wasn't responsible, I would have the opportunity to help her get there. I didn't know how, but I knew it would happen. The message was undeniable.

Quite a few years later, after I had a family of my own, I made a couple new friends that aided me on my path to energy healing. One was going through some intense emotional issues. The other knew how to help those issues. This friend told me that she did something called The Body Code and Rapid-Eye Movement therapy. I had no idea what those things were, but she said she helped people with emotional problems. I told my struggling friend this and encouraged her to go see "the Body Code Lady".

She wanted me to go with her, so I obliged. I was not prepared for the life-altering shock this simple decision had in my life.

From my upbringing, if you said the word "holistic" I scoffed. That term, along with "all-natural" and "organic" were just ploys to scare us into spending more money on things that didn't really work. But during my first session, this woman pushed on my out-stretched arm and told me I had something called a "trapped emotion" in my neck. She then ran a magnet over my head and told me it was gone....and that was it. She repeated the process a couple more times and then sent me on my way. I won't lie. My first thought was, "Is this witchcraft?" While later I learned that it wasn't, it sure seemed like it to me at the time! The thing was, we worked on this pain in my neck that I had for about ten years. After that session that pain subsided greatly. I was also feeling emotionally ten pounds lighter.

And so, still very skeptical but intrigued, I read the Emotion Code book by Dr. Bradley Nelson. So much was swimming through my mind as I read my first introduction to energy healing and what it was. What I read seemed so unbelievable but so interest-ing at the same time. The inner-child in me grew more and more excited because in a way, everything made so much sense and it was miraculous. But the jaded grown-up in me kept interjecting disbelieving thoughts in my mind.

"This is too good to be true". "Life does not work this way". "Healing can't be this simple". "This has SCAM written all over it". "Even if it can work, it's probably by some evil force and not of God".

I remember getting on my knees and asking with a sincere heart if the things I read in the Emotion Code were true. It took so much courage and strength to pray about it, because at that time I was so afraid of being wrong. I was afraid that I would get an angry answer: "How could you even ask such a question, of course it's not good!" But I knew I could not proceed learning this unless I felt confirmation that it was right. So I asked. And I felt unmistakable peace enter my heart. From that moment on, I knew I had stumbled onto something amazing.

I started slowly. I made my skinny and unhappy 15-year-old cat, Muffin, my first test-subject. The poor thing was my best friend till I moved away to college. And when I came back I found out that the sinus problems I had suffered with all my life were because I was allergic to cats! So I had to distance myself from her which caused her to become hardened and anti-social. As an experiment, I decided to try my own hand at this energy healing thing, and I released a few emotions from my cat. This was the first time I saw energy healing make a difference because of my own work. Muffin became a different cat overnight. Everyone noticed. She was suddenly much more social, playful and friendly.

Even after feeling the effects of energy healing in my neck, and seeing what it did to my cat, I was still very timid to approach my mother about this. Any time we even suggested her pain was because of emotions, we could have cut the tension with a knife. But this time, my approach would be different. This time, to have illness be emotionally-based didn't mean that it was just in her head, but that there were legitimate reasons causing her pain. Not only that, but there was something we could DO about them! To my relief, my mother didn't get upset with me when I introduced her to the Emotion Code. She said she would allow me to try it, but we both were still very dubious about the whole thing. While we wanted this to be successful, we were afraid we would end up throwing it on the pile of failed remedies.

My husband only knew my mother as an intense sufferer of disease, and, while he was always supportive of me exploring energy healing, he was extremely unconvinced of its validity. He would tell me, "I will believe in what you do once I see your mom out of bed for four days in a row."

By that year's Christmas, I sold my husband on Emotional healing. Not only was my mother up for four days, but she continued to be up for much longer than that. Although we are still working on her road to complete recovery, she is up and living life so much fuller than ever before. It is amazing to watch as she improves with each session and feels more healthy, strong and happy each time. Where before, she couldn't take three steps out of bed before falling over, she now travels to see her grandkids quite a lot and is able to enjoy spending time with them. After 20 years of searching, we finally found a miracle. The rainbow is a sign of miraculous promise. The rainbows I saw years before were a sign that my plea for my mother to be healed would be answered in a miraculous way.

My hope is that my story can give you hope. No matter how long or painful your suffering has been, there is an answer out there for you. Healing can be so simple. Christ-centered energy healing proves this to be true. But it is so hard for some of us to accept it being simple. Here are my tips if you are finding yourself in a similar situation like mine:

1. Just do it. The biggest hurdle for me was to take the actions first. I remember trying to get an undeniable, "YES, this is your course" endorsement from God before I was willing to give it my all. I had a fear of being wrong. I didn't want to ever be wrong. But that answer didn't come. It was only *after* I decided that I was going to be an energy healer, and I truly felt inside that it was what I wanted to do, that I got my personal endorsement from our Heavenly Father that it was pleasing to him that I do this work.

2. Don't let the critics get you down. Wikipedia, WebMD and other energy healing critics scoff at energy healing, saying

that results are just a coincidence or the placebo effect at best. I've been doing this professionally for two years now, working with about 300 clients. If all the successful results we've seen were just coincidences, then coincidences happen a whole heck of a lot more than I ever thought they could!

What about the placebo effect? Many doctors and scientists have the hardest time accepting that we can heal solely with the power of our minds. However, belief is strong. It has been said that faith is the strongest force on this earth. I believe that is true. The problem skeptics have about energy healing is that it is through our faith, belief, or intent that we are healed. It sounds like a nice story, but something that stays right there, in a story. It's not real life. I find it funny that whatever follows the terms "reality check" or "in the real world", is always intended to bring us down. Well, I say in the real world, healing was meant to be simple. Healing only became complicated when we started relying wholly on the science of western medicine to do it. There is nothing wrong with much of western medicine; in fact we have it to thank for many medical advancements. But in many ways, it has made us forget about the natural ways our bodies heal. My mother has taken pill after pill, done procedure after procedure, with little to no—or in some cases worse—results. Just a few sessions of "believing negative-energy out of the body" has done more for my mother in her healing than years of the best advancements in western medicine. However, it is good to note that even though the placebo effect and energy healing may be related, energy healing is much more than that. We see it work on babies and animals all the time, suggesting that there is more at play than our conscious mind believing the treatment will work.

3. Finally, don't get caught up in all the marketing. Healers are good at what they do. However, to many of us, marketing isn't one of our strong suits. Honestly, this is something

that bugs me about the energy healing world. All healing modalities are very keen to market their best, most successful stories. After reading all of the books and websites out there, you may get excited and feel that all of your woes and worries will be cured in one session. In a way, this kind of marketing helps. Again, it goes back the importance of belief. If you honestly believe and accept your problems will go away in one session, there is a better possibility that is true. To a very large extent, we create our reality. On the other hand, many, many times, there is just too much going on under the surface of your problems that one, or even a few sessions, just won't cut it.

You will see on the internet or in a book how Jane was swimming in debt, making no money with very little prospects. To her remarkable surprise, after just one session, she was promoted with a high pay-raise in her job the very next day. Yes, it is remarkable, and yes, we see results like this all the time. What the success story doesn't tell you is that Jane was also working on her arthritis problem and while it is improving, it's been 10 sessions and they still haven't completely resolved the issue.

I personally have seen people clear eczema issues after just a few sessions releasing trapped emotions, while other people with eczema are still trying to clear it after 10 sessions. Energy healing is amazing. But don't get carried away by all the hype. It still takes work and perseverance at times. Life was meant to be enjoyable and good...not problem-free. You are not going to get all of your problems healed in a couple of sessions. No, you will probably never get through all of your problems in this lifetime. But it will continually get better. You will learn things about yourself, you never knew before...remarkable things! Your life will become more peaceful, rewarding and full—not problem free, (what's the fun in that, anyway?). But you will become stronger and more capable to handle those challenges that keep coming our way.

Energy healing gives us the tools to handle life's challenges with more hope, belief and quicker healing.

Christ-centered energy healing is a wonderful tool. It is an answer to many prayers. It is simple, it is beautiful and it is based on true principles about how our bodies work and the laws they are governed by. Enjoy your journey; it only gets more fascinating from here!

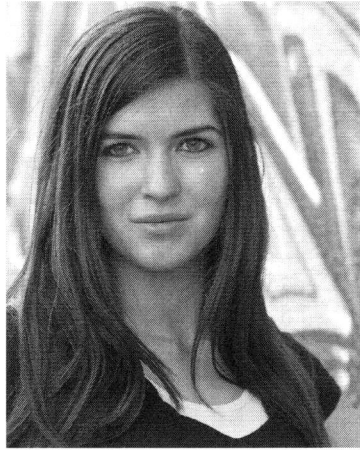

JAMIE JENSEN

Jamie is a happy mother of three and married to her very best friend. She is an outdoor enthusiast, master foot zoner, instructor, blogger, presenter and author of The Living Diet. *She is the owner and founder of* Good Health is Happiness; Integrated Healing Arts and Institute.

Foot zoning and the healing arts have been a great part of her own journey in healing naturally from chronic disease. Today she is disease free and living life well. She has great faith in the tender mercies that are given from God through these great tools like foot zoning, the healing arts and energy medicine.

www.goodhealthishappiness.com

I came to a knowledge of the healing arts and energy medicine a few years after I was diagnosed with Chronic Kidney Disease.

I had a new baby, and any new mom can attest that it is life-changing to have a child, but especially the first!

My baby didn't sleep through the night until after he turned a year old. I was tired...unbelievably tired, all the time! It was all I could do to get out of bed to do necessary tasks like getting the baby out of bed, changing his diaper, getting him fed—you know, taking care of basic needs. While I did this, I usually would lay down anywhere I could, just to get a break from exhaustion. At the time, I thought this was normal from having a non-sleeping baby and all.

One day, it came to light! I went on a vacation with my mom and baby to see my grandma. My mom quickly realize, after seeing how extremely tired I was and watching my need to repeatedly lay down that this was not just a "non-sleeping" baby problem. She knew better—she had raised a few of her own after all!

When we returned from grandma's, I made a trip to the ol' doc and had everything tested. Honestly, I expected the results to be normal! But then I got "the call" from the doctor's office saying I needed to come back in, results were abnormal. I was still in doubt and kind of assumed it wasn't anything really serious,' because really, that never happens to me, right?! Well, I went in and WOW, this was serious—Chronic Kidney Disease, or CKD. My kidney function was pretty much rock-bottom, and my body was full of toxins. This was causing the extreme fatigue! How did this happen? I was such a healthy person! I ate well, I was young, fit and somehow still found myself plagued with disease! How? I not only had this disease, but serious depression crept in. Something that someone who has never experienced could never fully understand the feeling of darkness and loneliness that comes with this. And worse, I hid the depression from my husband and family. I wasn't me.

I thought about the options I had for treatment, I prayed and knew that for me I wasn't ready to do the usual thing. I told my doctor I wanted to try a more natural route first. He only agreed if I would come in for regular testing to make sure my kidneys were actually improving and not getting worse or just maintaining their current state. My doctor suggested a couple supplements that might aid in the process, and off I went on my journey to learn much more than I ever expected! A few days later I was introduced to essential oils from a great friend, and also met with a health coach and changed just a couple more things that what I was doing: alkaline water, fresh green drinks (without any sugar or artificial sugar!), Redmond real salt, chlorophyll, fresh herbs and a major revamp of my personal hygiene products. I had to get rid of all things chemically unnatural, even if it was on the outside. I had to make sure I had all my bases covered so I was giving my body an environment worthy of letting the healing begin.

The healing began! It was like spring had finally started after the darkest, most bitter winter. Slowly, but surely it was happening, Tests were done repeatedly and miraculously my body was healing! After a year and a half, my kidneys were in the normal range again. My body was healing so much, but every once in a while, I would still feel jolts of serious pain through my kidneys. I knew I hadn't found complete healing yet. It wasn't until three years later that I unintentionally found a healing therapy called foot zoning that my health problems resolved completely. At the time, I was unaware of anything that could help the body heal that wasn't a supplement or pill of some kind.

I had a friend mention a couple times over the course of two years about her sister who did this "foot" thing. Then one day my friend called and told me her sister was here from Hawaii for just a few hours and I needed to meet her and get a foot zone. Knowing my friend, I knew I needed to do what she said right then. So I met Stephanie for the first time after hearing mention of her for two years and got my feet "done". I had hope, but was a skeptic to say the least before the session.

I have to say, she told me things about my body she could NEVER have guessed, ever! Including a weak physical connection between the heart and brain. Little did she know, I had landed in the emergency room a few years prior for unexplained heart problems that were related to unexplained low potassium levels and a weak electrical impulse from the brain to the heart. Wow! She is a very in-tune Christ-centered practitioner. I know the heart problems and CKD were correlated for a long time running but didn't realize it 'til later. I had never experienced any alternative therapy or energy medicine and it was different, but good! Stephanie also made mention of releasing an emotion of feeling overwhelmed. I didn't think I had that emotion at the time. I thought it was odd too, but about a day after the foot zone, it was so noticeable, I couldn't help but give credit to the foot zone.

All of a sudden, it was like a weight was lifted from me all the way down to my soul. I had a clarity in my mind and heart, almost as if I had been living in an overcast world and suddenly the sunlight broke through to show what the world was like with real sunshine burning through. Fear was gone from me and peace filled its place. This was healing at a level that I had never experienced before. It was real! It was different! The physical aspect was finally met with mental, emotional and spiritual healing. It is Christ-centered energy healing!

I decided the next week to go through her trial foot zone program she created online that was completely long-distance. I would be one of the first "guinea pigs" to see if distance learning for foot zoning and energy work was possible. I would be learning remotely; while she was in Hawaii and I in Utah. Not really knowing a lot about foot zoning or energy medicine at the time, but having faith in the prompting to continue learning, I learned, and very well at that! I know now there is hope for those needing Christ-centered, faith-driven education for foot zoning and energy medicine across the world, because now it is possible to reach across the world with inspired education remotely!

Let's just say that one foot zone changed my life and health forever, as well as all the lives it has touched through me.

This whole healing process was a God-given gift. I know these years of hardship and learning with my health were truly a blessing from God—a blessing in disguise, a blessing to know that I am His, that his plans are much bigger than my plans. I know He was with me through it all, even when I felt alone. I know we are never alone! In our darkest of moments we have not been forgotten, only our faith tried.

I continue to study anything healing or preventative and thank Heavenly Father for my knowledge and experience. We can have hope! God is with you, He is with us, His plans are greater than our own, to truly teach us in our own unique ways. I hope my story can bring even a glimmer of hope to someone else fighting their fight. You are never alone.

You are worth the journey!

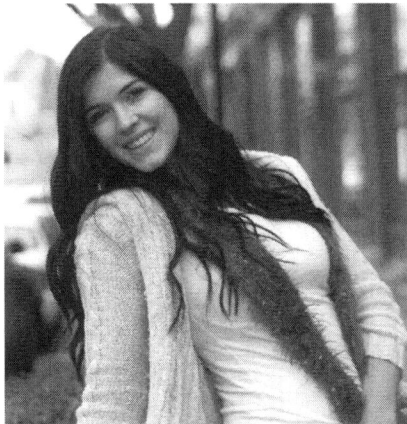

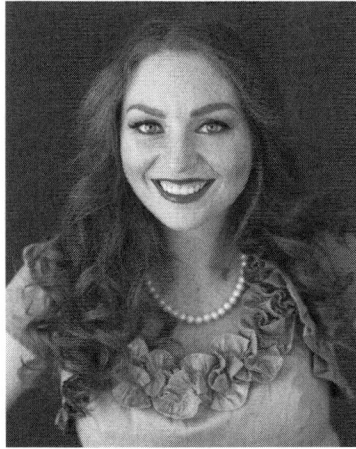

MELISSA EGGERTSEN

Melissa Eggertsen is a Licensed Massage Therapist, certified reflexologist, birth educator, yoga instructor, and energy intuitive. Knowledge and experience combine with clairvoyance as she uses her God-given gifts to educate and serve those around her. Being a mother of three young children who enrich and enhance her life is one of her greatest treasures. Melissa and her husband David are Certified Parenting Mentors with Teaching Self Government. Melissa is dedicated to continuing her education and helping others to do the same. Teaching is her passion and she is a sought-after presenter and mentor.

perceptivehealing.com
melissa@perceptivehealing.com

At six years old, I remember going up to a gentleman I hardly knew and telling him how beautiful his wife was. I could see her red hair blowing in the wind, the deep wrinkles in her face, her sharp blue eyes. In great detail, I described to the man how she looked and the words she was whispering to me. He started sobbing, and explained that his wife had passed away just four weeks earlier. Her image was so vivid to me, I was surprised that he didn't also see it. His tears were overwhelming to me, and I was frightened by the depth of the experience. Was there something wrong with me? Why could I see things that others could not?

When I was nine, my best friend told me that her parents were getting a divorce. She was confused, and I asked her if I could look directly in her eyes to show her Heavenly Father's love for her. As I stared into her pupils, I felt the questions she was asking. Her eyes reflected back to me all of the answers, though when I started speaking the words her spirit was dictating to me, she turned away. There was so much pain, and I think she was afraid of what would surface. Instead, she decided to hide, unwilling even to receive the love that God was sending her. At the time, I took it personally and felt that I was being rejected. I determined that I must not be a safe person, as I couldn't even help my best friend.

As a child, I didn't realize that the things I saw and felt were different from what others experienced. I didn't want to be different. I was afraid something was wrong with me and decided that this "gift" of seeing was hurting people. I didn't tell anyone about it, for fear of rejection. I even asked God to take this awareness away from me. It was too hard to be able to see and feel the thoughts and emotions of another person, particularly if they were seeking to avoid the very things I was bringing to the surface. Heavenly Father answered my prayers and took away my gift of seeing with my spiritual eyes.

Crushing news came just before my twelfth birthday. I knew that my parents had temporarily separated, but I was told that they had every intention of getting together after a six month period. As I was visiting my father one afternoon, I looked at a calendar he had on the wall. I noticed that just three weeks away, hand-written in my father's writing were the words, "my wedding". I was struck with confusion as I turned to him and asked what the words meant. He explained that the paperwork for divorce had been finalized last month, but neither of my parents had the heart to tell me. He had already made arrangements to marry another woman, though I didn't get so much as an announcement. Loneliness and fear enveloped me as my mother told me we would be moving right away from the only home I had ever known in Las Vegas, NV to a small condominium in Provo, UT so that she could get her doctorate degree from Brigham Young University.

During the next several years, my mother became my closest friend. My other siblings were grown and gone, and it was just the two of us. We would share a bed and every night we would give each other back rubs. Every time I put my hands on her, I felt all of her pain and suffering. In my own body, in the exact location I was touching her, I felt precisely what she was feeling both physically and emotionally. Though the spiritual gift of sight had left me, I was given the gift to feel. There was so much pain, shame, doubt, tension, feelings of unworthiness, and abandonment I could feel in my mother when I placed my hands on her. I wanted so badly to take these horrific feelings from her, so I did. I put all of the tension and aching within my own body. In time, I started feeling all of the same emotions my mother had been struggling with for years. It was heavy for a little girl to handle. There was no separation between her emotions and my own as I felt loneliness, shame, and inadequacy. I struggled finding friends, and having relationships with any sort of depth. And of course, I couldn't tell my mother of the feelings I was experiencing or she would feel guilty which would trigger even more shame and unworthiness. So, in order to stop the cycle, I had to protect her. I had to take the pain and keep quiet.

I both yearned for and feared deep connection and friendships. I so badly wanted validation and safety but feared that my own pains would burden others, or that I wouldn't have the capacity to take on another's aches and suffering with my already saturated capacity and heavy load.

As time went on, I began to isolate myself from others. Throughout middle school and high school, I didn't develop many friendships, and had a difficult time relating to my peers. My life was full of secrets. Secrets about the circumstances of my parents' divorce, secrets about how I was feeling on the inside, even secrets about where I lived. My mother feared my father finding us, so no one was to know the exact location of our home. I didn't have anyone I could share all of my shame with, and it started to fester like a wound within me.

I went to college, but nothing seemed to change. Not really. At some point, I decided that it must be better to feel nothing at all than all of the pain that surrounded me. For years I tried to escape my own life, and severe depression set in. Sleeping a solid 18 hours a day became my new norm. I ate very little and would rarely leave the house. I started to become numb to all emotions. More than anything, I wanted to unexist. Waking up was a painful reality, so I decided to overdose on all of the pills I could find in the hopes that I may never wake up.

I remember being in the hospital bed as they pumped my stomach with charcoal to rid my body of the toxins I had ingested. My roommate had found me and knew something was wrong. She found the evidence, forced me to wake up, and drove me to the hospital herself.

My family was in shock. How had they not known how badly I had been suffering? How had I been able to isolate myself so successfully? Questions left unanswered for them. By this time, my mother realized the gravity of the situation and immediately enrolled me as a resident of The Bridge Recovery Center, an intensive recovery program in Southern Utah.

In the few weeks I spent in the recovery facility, things started shifting dramatically for me. I was the youngest participant in the program and was able to see a clear vision of where I would be in 10, 20, and even 30 years from that point if I continued on the path I was taking. This facility incorporated both Western Medicine practices and Holistic Healthcare techniques to facilitate whole-body healing on a core level. I started noticing changes immediately with a whole foods diet, daily yoga, meditation, exercise, massages, chiropractic care, acupuncture, counseling and group therapies that I received. My mind was cleansed of toxic thoughts, and I was encouraged to start dreaming and creating the life I longed for.

This healing environment was the best medicine I could have conjured up. I learned to love and embrace myself, to share the secrets I had been hiding, and to become a seeker of truth. I realized I had been listening to lies, and the programming of my mind was running a long chain of false beliefs. Ironically, where I had previously thought that I had been easing my mother's burdens by taking her pains, I began to realize that I had been doubling the load for each of us by ignoring the greatest healing power in the universe: the atonement of Jesus Christ.

Through my recovery process, I was taught to turn to my Savior, and I chose to plead with him to take away the burdens I had placed on myself. I remember asking for room in my heart to receive all of the blessings I knew He wanted to send me. I took a leap of faith by opening up my heart.

Exactly five weeks from the time I had tried to take my own life and ended up in a hospital bed, I once again found myself on the edge of existence, this time not of my doing. Part-way through my therapy program, I had driven to Provo for my brother's wedding. On the way back to Southern Utah, I was in a devastating accident where my car was completely totaled. Having rolled all the way across the freeway facing oncoming traffic, every corner of my car was dented, with glass shattered into millions of pieces. My life literally flashed before my eyes. I recall shutting my eyes tight, afraid to open them because I knew I would be dead. The woman that opened my car door was as shocked as I was to find myself alive and without a single scratch. Not a drop of blood or a broken bone. It was at this point that I became absolutely certain that there is a God and my plans cannot thwart His. From attempting to take my own life to facing certain death, yet untouched, I know that God is master and creator.

This experience gave me clarity and courage. I determined to dedicate my life to the Lord with unwavering faith. My life was no accident, and I was ready to discover its purpose. I remembered the spiritual gifts I had been given as a child and prayed in humility that they would return to me. My prayers were again answered, and I was given the gift of touch and of connecting with individuals eye to eye, soul to soul.

I connected with my mother once again, opening up my heart, showing her that we could both give our burdens to Christ. As we sought the healing of the atonement of Christ, our burdens were lightened and our hearts freed. We were each blessed with the gift of finding and marrying the men of our dreams. I feel so blessed to have the support and love of my incredible husband, David, so that together we can build and create our dreams as we help others recognize and embrace their life purpose.

With the support of my husband, my passion to help others find their purpose and reclaim their lives was ignited. I felt that I should enroll in massage therapy school to gain additional tools to compliment my spiritual gifts. Upon graduating, I felt strongly that I needed to continue learning about energy work. I was hesitant at first because of my desire to learn only from individuals who honored and shared my same belief system. I was not interested in

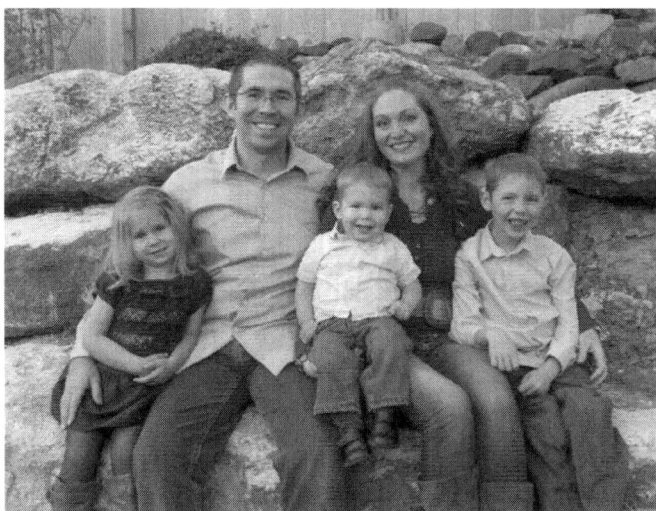

proclaiming myself as a Healer; I know that the only true Healer is Jesus Christ. I simply want to help facilitate His love and be a conduit of His light.

In time, mentors came who were able to teach me more about my spiritual gifts by accessing the healing power of the atonement. Now, passing that knowledge to others is one of my greatest joys. I absolutely love teaching classes and mentoring groups and individuals. My greatest desire is to be a conduit of Christ's love and to inspire individuals to connect to Jesus Christ so that they might receive the same healing I have experienced, illuminating the path to our Savior.

My purpose in sharing this story with you is to give you hope, wherever you are. Whether you are unsure of your spiritual gifts, or are aware of them and are looking for a mentor to help you further develop them, keep moving forward. You will be strengthened and fortified as you take action. God needs you in his army to fight for truth and right. Throughout my journey, this quote gave me courage and strength, and inspiration. I hope you feel the same.

"Our deepest fear is not that we are inadequate. Our deepest fear is that we are powerful beyond measure. It is our light, not our darkness that most frightens us. We ask ourselves, 'Who am I to be brilliant, gorgeous, talented, fabulous?' Actually, who are you not to be? You are a child of God. Your playing small does not serve the world. There is nothing enlightened about shrinking so that other people won't feel insecure around you. We are all meant to shine, as children do. We were born to make manifest the glory of God that is within us. It's not just in some of us; it's in everyone. And as we let our own light shine, we unconsciously give other people permission to do the same. As we are liberated from our own fear, our presence automatically liberates others."

—*Marianne Williamson*

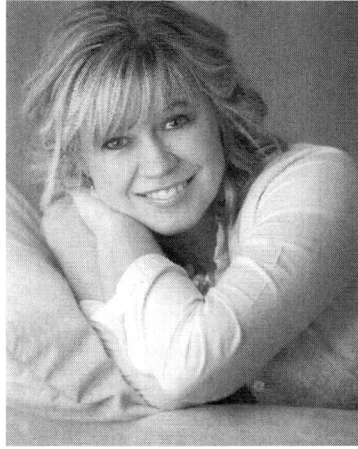

ROBIN JOHNSON

Robin fell in love with the man she later married when she was 13 years old. They have been married for 28 years and have four amazing children that are the joy of their lives!

Robin is a Reiki master/teacher and has taught over 80 Reiki classes now. She loves to empower people with this simple gift for healing and also hosts an annual Reiki Retreat. She became a Heart Centered Therapist and is amazed at the power of the heart for healing.

She is a professional photographer as well. Whether she is behind a camera, doing Reiki, or working with the heart, she sees the best in others and helps them see it in themselves.

When I think about sharing my healing journey, I feel so much gratitude. It is just a story to me now—it is no longer my life. If there is one thing I hope to convey, it is that regardless of what you are struggling with, there is a path that will take you beyond your pain. My life experiences and what

I came to believe about them affected every day of my life until I started a path to healing. I praise God for that journey.

I grew up in a home filled with people. There were eight kids along with my mom and dad. We lived out in the country, so nature was my playground and my haven. Our home life was pleasant. Despite the fact that there were ten of us, it was always calm. For the most part, everyone was kind. It was peaceful, but things had to fit in a pretty tight box emotionally. If we were too loud or crazy, we were told to settle down. Crying made my dad extremely uncomfortable, and so we learned to hide our tears. We never said, "I love you," because that would be too personal. Everything had to be in perfect order. On the surface everything was "fine."

Underneath the facade, there was trouble in my parents' marriage that I wasn't consciously aware of. One night when my father was gone, my mom gathered all the kids together to tell us they were separating. She explained why, but I didn't understand words like "adultery" and "infidelity." I was 10 years old. I don't know how long it was before I understood what was going on. I just remember my friend telling me at school one day that she knew my parents got divorced because my dad loved another woman. I was devastated.

I was 12 when the divorce finally went through. There was no fanfare. No arguing. No decisions for us to make. My parents kept it simple for the kids. My dad moved out and we all stayed with my mom. We never talked about the divorce as a family again.

Life went on. Our home stayed calm. The house felt different, but no one talked about any of it. I didn't know what to do with all the emotion inside of me. I had been a daddy's girl. I used to shingle roofs with him. He was an artist, and I would watch him paint just to be near him. I looked like him. I had the same gifts as him. And then... he was just gone.

I had always been a bright light—in fact my mom called me her "little sunshine"—but that light started to fade, and I began to struggle with waves of depression. I had been a straight A student but found myself not caring much about school. Something would trigger me and I would spend three or four days spiraling downward. There was no stopping it. Once I hit the bottom, I would spend three or four days climbing out of the hole I was in. It seemed to happen at least once a month. It was a rollercoaster ride.

As a 13-year-old, I had fallen in love with Andrew Johnson, a foreign exchange student living with my best friend's family. We both dated other people during my high school years. After my first year at BYU, he started asking me out. He was 25 and ready to get married; I was 19 and barely survived my first year of college. I could tell he was getting serious, and so I started praying for guidance. I received an undeniable witness from God that he was the one I should marry. I was thrilled and terrified at the same time!

The closer we got, the more anxiety I had about our relationship. I had loved him for six years and never in my wildest dreams thought he would be mine—and now the chance was right in front of me. I was in summer semester, and I remember sitting in class one day just thinking about getting married. I nearly fainted, I was so scared.

I went to a counselor. He asked a list of questions about Andrew: Would he support me? Did he treat me right? Was I attracted to him? Did I trust him? Everything got a resounding yes! And then he asked if I wanted to get married. I looked away and said, "I don't know." He explained that what was happening to me happens to many children in divorced homes. They get in relationships and get right to the point of commitment, then back out because they are scared. He said, "Andrew sounds like a wonderful man, and I can tell you love him. You get to decide when you have the courage to face your fears."

I left the office aware of the effects that my parents' divorce had on me for the first time. I didn't realize that was where the fear and anxiety were coming from. I was angry at my dad. I knew I didn't want to lose the man I loved. Andrew later proposed, and I found the courage to accept. We were married that Christmas, and I was delighted to find how fun and fulfilling marriage could be to a wonderful man.

We moved to Arizona when Andrew finished graduate school and began our little family. Once I had a child, I began to struggle again, seeing my dad with a different perspective. How could he leave his children behind? My depression seemed exaggerated with each additional child that was born. Being a mom of young kids left me little time to nurture myself or sort things out. I would see other new moms that seemed happy and had their life together. I kept up on the surface, but inside I was sinking lower and lower into depression. I wondered—did everyone fake happiness, or were there people who were truly happy every single day? My husband seemed happy every day. My friends did too. I couldn't believe it was possible. What was wrong with me? I felt that happiness would never be part of my daily life.

About this time, my friend Julie learned Reiki. She called and asked me if she could practice on me. I had no idea what it was, and she explained that it would balance the energy and emotion in my body. I needed help, so I went in for the session and was amazed at the experience. She could feel where I was holding on to negative emotions and helped me release them. She could tell that part of me had shut down, and she helped me open up again. She felt the barrage of negative thoughts I had about myself in my head and cleared them out. When we were done, I felt like a new person! I felt like someone had pushed a reset button on my soul, and I had a clean slate to start again. It was incredible!

My sessions with Julie continued. For the first time in my life I felt like there was help to get me through those times when things started sliding downhill emotionally. Julie was gifted, intuitive, and centered in Christ. She continued to do Reiki for me and my children while we lived in Arizona.

When our youngest son was 18 months old, we decided to move back to Utah. My father was dying of Parkinson's disease and our kids were growing up without any extended family around. In Utah, they had 24 cousins and wonderful aunts and uncles that we wanted to be part of their lives. We said goodbye to our Arizona friends and moved home.

Going home meant going back to issues. Seeing my dad's health failing and the thought of him leaving me again was more than I could bear. He couldn't talk about emotional issues, and so nothing was ever said or resolved.

I didn't have Julie nearby to help me anymore. I remember at one point feeling like I was done trying to cope with the emotional rollercoaster of my life. I just wanted a pill to make me feel better. My sister referred me to an energy worker named Kirt who did tapping and emotional release techniques. During our sessions, I opened up about my life and my healing journey continued. I remember once telling Kirk about the week-long emotional spiral that seemed to come every month. By then, I had been experiencing it for over 20 years. We went back to my childhood and realized that the divorce happened the same time that I matured physically as a young woman. My monthly cycle began just when I saw my mom going through a divorce. I felt like she was the victim in the circumstance, and I associated being a woman with being a victim. Each month as that cycle came, I was pulled back into that emotional trap of feeling bad about myself. When that became conscious for me, Kirk did his work to clear the issue. I was completely surprised to see that the monthly cycle of depression never happened again.

I couldn't believe that emotion stored in the body could create that pattern every month. Clearing the emotional trigger within my body cleared the response in my heart and mind. It was a miracle! I have had many healing sessions since that time.

I learned how to do Reiki and found that not only can I use it to help others, I can use it for myself! Rather than waiting for something to trigger my fears and depression cycle, I check in with myself at night and see if something feels off. If something is wrong, I can balance it out and go to bed with a clean emotional slate every night. I also learned Heart Centered Therapy, which has a profound effect on healing us with the wisdom of the heart at a soul level.

I know myself enough to know that I will always be sensitive to emotional balance. I have a gentle heart and it is easy for me to get hurt. I get to be responsible for that. I don't watch violent or scary movies. I listen to good music. I have an energy session of some sort every six weeks or so to help me stay on track. I do things that bring energy and light into my life—I eat healthy, I exercise and enjoy nature, I read the scriptures, pray daily, and attend the temple. All of these things strengthen me emotionally and spiritually when I do them.

In all of this healing, I have come closer to Christ. When I could let go of all that darkness inside of me, there was more room for His light. I have learned the power of the atonement as I was able to truly forgive my dad for all that happened. He passed away ten years ago and I can honestly say I love him and look forward to the day we will meet again.

I found a scripture that has been a great teacher to me: "For God hath not given us the spirit of fear, but of power and of love and of a sound mind" (2 Timothy 1:7). This scripture helps me identify when I am getting off track. If I am giving in to fear and anxiety, I know I am disconnecting from God and my faith. I focus on holding my personal power, feeling God's unconditional love, clearing my mind of anxiety and doubt, and trusting God. It is powerful to realize God does not EVER give us the spirit of fear! I truly believe that God wants us to be happy and I am grateful to say I live happy every day. It is something I used to only dream about feeling.

I am so thankful for the opportunities I have now in my life to teach Reiki and empower others with this same healing gift. I am so grateful for Heart Centered Therapy that truly helps my clients get to the bottom of their issues and clear them from their life—like Kirk did for me. I find such joy as I work with clients, helping them find room for the Savior in their heart as we call upon the atonement and release negative and unwanted emotions. My greatest joy is helping people release their traumas so they can find Christ and live in the truth of who they are.

And as for my 28 years of marriage? My sweet companion Andrew is my best friend. He is my anchor in the storms of life. He is honest, funny, trustworthy, supportive and kind. We LOVE time together. We work hard at our marriage and the rewards are so fulfilling!

I am blessed for the lessons my journey has taught me. I pray that your journey will be filled with the light of truth, the love of our Savior and hope for healing.

Sending you my love!

Robin

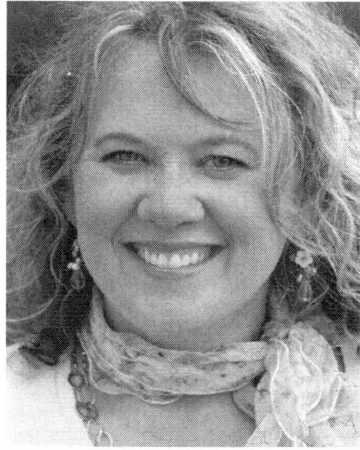

LaurieKae Banks

LaurieKae V. Banks has worked in the wellness industry for over two decades. She loves to travel and study history wherever she goes. LaurieKae is a professional speaker and mentor with a solution-based focus. She takes an eclectic approach to coaching and is certified in many different healing modalities. LaurieKae has given birth to eight fabulous individuals and has been blissfully married to Sam Banks Sr. for over 23 years. LaurieKae has developed her strong testimony of Jesus Christ as a member of the Church of Jesus Christ of Latter Day Saints. We invite you to go to www.LaurieKae.com to learn more.

As far back as I can remember, I have desired to know the mysteries of God and his creations. But I have wondered, is it possible to comprehend the wondrousness of his works? Can we even begin to understand the workings of the human body, or the universe? Is it really true what it says in Luke 11:9 "Ask, and it shall be given you; seek, and ye shall find; knock, and it shall be opened unto you"? Through my personal journey of searching and questioning, I have come to understand that He does answer prayers. The secrets of the universe are open to us, but we must begin by knocking. We must begin with a desire to know.

I remember giving my dad a back rub when I was about three years old. He told me I was the best back rubber. I took that lesson, and grew up feeling some element of pride in my "massage giving skills". As an adult, I decided to become a massage therapist.

I enjoyed learning about the workings of the human anatomy and how each one of the body systems works together. Massage therapy came naturally to me. I learned I have an instinct for massage therapy. As I work on different areas of the body, I almost feel as though the muscles are speaking to me. I become aware of emotions that may be stored in a muscle. If I close my eyes, I can see the way the muscles intersect and connect. I learned so much.

Then, the classes I was taking took a new turn. They introduced the concept of energy healing, chakras and meridians. I was highly skeptical, especially when they said chakras were like tornadoes, vortexes of energy protruding from the fronts and backs of our bodies. I was not open to this. I was convinced this was the biggest bunch of hullaballoo I had ever heard. I was uncomfortable giving credence to something so few people could validate. I wondered how anyone could buy into these concepts. God was being patient with me.

Being a Christian all of my life, I had gained a respect for the body as a gift from our Heavenly Father. The more I did bodywork, the more I saw this to be true. The body is not just a gift; it is a sacred gift. The fact that others come to me for bodywork is a sacred honor. Before each appointment, I pray to be an instrument in the Lord's hands for the person on whom I am about to work. One day, I was working on a woman who was under a lot of stress. As I worked on her, I closed my eyes for a moment. Suddenly, in my mind, I saw the room I was working in. I saw three people standing near the door as though they were on security detail. It occurred to me that they were guardian angels for the woman I was working on.

This surprised and shocked me. I believe in guardian angels. I had heard of them all of my life. I have family members who have seen their own angels as they have faced some scary situations. With all of this, I did not imagine I would ever see someone else's guardian angels. Seeing angels started to happen quite frequently. It became rare for me to work on someone without seeing their guardian angels. Sometimes there were several angels; sometime there was only one.

I wanted to share this with some of those I was closest to. I chose carefully who I was going to open up to about this. I chose to share it separately with each of my parents and two of my siblings. Each of them had a different reaction. Each was surprised, and some of were extremely apprehensive. A few of them told me, "God doesn't work like that," and others asked if I had been ill. One of them even said that I was out of line in mentioning it to them because if it had really happened, I wouldn't be sharing it with them. It would have been too sacred to share. My mother suggested that I take some time to ask myself some questions about what I was experiencing and to record it in a private journal, which I did. But they all started to treat me a little differently. I didn't like it.

I put bodywork on hold. I packed everything having anything to do with massage or bodywork away into storage. I didn't work on anyone for years other than a few very close friends and family. I no longer prayed before I worked on someone. I made a conscious effort to not experience anything anyone would deem unusual. I did not want to have an unfavorable experience.

Years passed. I ran into a former neighbor and close friend who had followed a similar path to mine. While neighbors, we had each started massage therapy school at the same time. We had attended the same church and had shared our testimonies multiple times with one another. I knew her to be a strong Christian woman with immense faith. Now, however, I saw her doing something that caused me great concern. She was teaching classes on crystals. I felt compelled to bring my concerns to her and help direct her back to truth. So I decided to attend her class.

I was expecting crystal ball divination type training, but it wasn't. The class was really just about the way different elements carry different electrical currents and how energy works differently with each stone. We learned each emotion we have carries a different energy with it, and crystals have the possibility of gently affecting these subtle energies within the body. It wasn't at all what I expected, and it prepared me for future experiences.

My brother had passed away less than three months before I took the class on crystals. He had been one of the family members with whom I had shared the guardian angels experience. He had not accepted that such things were possible. The sharing of my experience with him changed our relationship which was never repaired. Months after his death, I was still struggling to function, and I was close to a breaking point. I decided I was no longer going to require God to work in a certain way for me. With a broken heart, I asked my Heavenly Father to answer my prayers however he saw fit to do so. This is when God graced me with a dream of my brother.

In my dream, my brother came to talk to me. He told me so many things that began to heal my heart. He explained that although he hadn't understood what I had tried to share with him, he did now. He was sorry about the way he had reacted. He then told me I was wrong to have given so much power to the words of those who had been critical. God had blessed me with these experiences, and I was dishonoring my Savior by stifling the gift that I had been given. I knew then that I needed to change and turn my heart back to God and away from the pride of the world. I was able to share with my brother once more how much I loved him and that missing him was almost more than I could bare. He told me that it is possible for all things to be healed through Jesus Christ and to have faith. I was reminded I would not be left alone. My mind went back to the guardian angels that I had been blessed to see with others. This experience was one of the most sacred and special gifts that I had ever been given. But still, the sadness lingered.

I ordered the least expensive crystal necklace I could find, which was a carnelian necklace on eBay. I was still worried about the judgment of others, so I put the necklace on just before bed making sure that my pj's and hair covered all of it. On the way to bed, I saw my four-year-old son.

"Mom," he asked, "Why are you all orange?"

Shocked, I looked down to see if he was referring to my necklace, but it was completely covered. "I don't know. What you are talking about?"

"You are orange all over you."

"Hmm. I don't know, Honey." I replied, and swiftly walked to my bedroom. My head was spinning just a little bit.

I let a few days pass before I asked, "Honey, remember the other night when you stopped me at bedtime and asked about why I was all orange?"

"Yes."

"Can you tell me what you were talking about?"

He told me that he had never seen me all orange before. In fact, I wasn't just all orange, even all of my dots were orange. My mind raced to find anything that would give me a foundation of what my son was talking about. I mentally reviewed what I vaguely remembered from those "hullaballoo" classes from years before. I asked him question after question over the next several days. My mind went often to the experience I had when I shared what I had seen with others. I desired my son to have a different experience, so I was cautious. He shared how he saw different colors on others and that the different colors reacted in different ways on the body. At one point, he was looking at my back and talking to me about the colors he was seeing there and they were moving. He said it looked like a tornado. My mind was blown. 'What in the world? A tornado? A vortex? Could it be that there was some validity to the "hullaballoo" that I poo-pooed so many years ago?'

It was during this period of time that my younger children were studying the solar system and my older children were studying atoms. In our family, God comes up in many of our conversations, even when we are studying the solar system and atoms. Somehow, I happened to see the diagrams side by side. They looked oddly similar. I had an epiphany. The Lord God, our creator, had created the largest systems, down to the smallest systems. Could it be that He follows patterns? If atoms are what make up us, could we have similar patterns in ourselves? It occurred to me that it was possible that the same energetic patterns could be running through us. To discard this possibility would be ignorant. It was like the Lord opened up a window of understanding to me. I began to get a glimpse of his greatness and wisdom.

This knowledge and awareness opened up my world for the study of patterns. These patterns are all around us, from the seasons to our heartbeats. What a wondrous place this world is. Like many others, I have a deep desire to understand the ways of the Lord. I recognize that I am only one person—a sinner in the eyes of

God—but I am also His daughter, a divine child of the Most High God. He is my Father in Heaven. I no longer believe the lie that says, "God doesn't work that way." I feel as the author of the song Amazing Grace, John Newton, "(I) was blind, but now I see." I know there is so much more for us to learn. I have found so much joy in discovering that I continue to be given more and more gifts. Being a good back rubber was just the beginning. I love being a mentor, a coach, a speaker, a healer, a mother, a wife and a friend. What a blessing to be an instrument in God's hands. Heavenly Father does answer prayers and the secrets of the universe are open to us if we ask. It all begins when we desire to know.

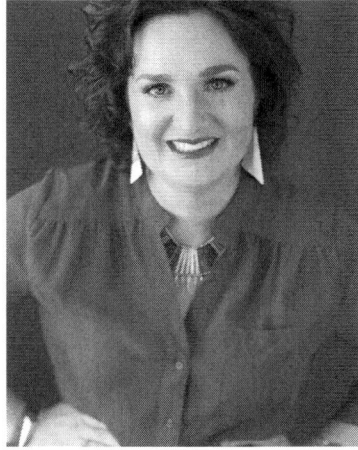

SASKIA STALLINGS

Saskia is a mother of seven and grandmother to two. She is a published author, social worker, Certified SimplyHealed™ Practitioner, mentor, speaker and lover of life. She lives her life with purpose and inspires others to do the same. She lives in St. George, Utah with her amazing husband and children. She enjoys laughing and connecting to her inner child. She believes it takes courage to heal, and that our life experiences are beautiful masterpieces as we step into our Divine Purpose. Her motto is "Embrace Your Purpose". She loves God, authenticity, vulnerability, courage, and people.

www.saskiaspeaks.com

One night as a little girl, I was lying in my bed. I was thinking of all the events of the day. I was feeling lost, scared, confused, but deep within my heart, I knew something: I was a Child of God, and I was special. I knew that God needed me for something great. At the time, I didn't know what, but I knew that no matter what, I must keep going in life.

Fifteen years old was the age I made the connection that I had been sexually abused. There was more than sexual abuse in my childhood, but this violation of my body and spirit had caused me the most turmoil. It was during that time that I received a beautiful confirmation from my Father in Heaven. I was to help people come out of darkness and into the light. I decided at that time that I wanted to be a social worker. It made sense to me, as my mom was recently divorced with nine children, and I saw the hope the women called social workers brought to us. I wanted to help people just like they did, so becoming a social worker seemed to be the way I would help others heal.

At 21 years of age I found myself a single mother. I had a one-year-old daughter, Echo, and a two-day-old baby boy, Draven. I was in the process of wanting a divorce, but not sure how to do it. I was very much alone and still suffering from my own childhood and the abuse that I endured in my marriage. Many events took place with the man I was married to at the time, including his being convicted of aggravated assault towards me that led to his imprisonment. It was during that time that I told myself when my baby was a year old, I was going back to school. And that's what I did. I pursued a degree in social work. My ex got out of prison, and due to my struggles of self-worth and personal value I allowed him into my life off and on. I was working and going to college and taking care of two little ones. I wanted them to have a relationship with their father. I wasn't in tune to my Heavenly Father and was merely surviving.

When my daughter was five years old, and I had two weeks left of college, I found out that my husband at the time, had sexually abused her. This was horrific for me. I stayed up all night long in turmoil, and the next morning I drove to his residence so I could get an address and report him. I had tried to report him the night before but without an address, they wouldn't take the report. He was convicted and ended up going to prison. I got a job as a social worker, and went on with my life dealing with children who were in deep pain. After finding out about the abuse of my daughter, I was in a low place. I thought no one would want us. I was 25 years old. My kids would act out and many times I'd go outside and shut the door and just cry, feeling so lost. Every time people from church came to visit me, I'd break down crying. I hurt so badly, my children hurt, and I didn't know what to do. I met a man during this time and he felt like a step up from what I was used to. I found myself pregnant with my 3rd child. This was a time of great shame for me. First, I was religious and this was against what I was taught as I was not married. Second, it wasn't even who I truly was.

And third, I was alone. I was so mean to myself that if anyone from church wanted to judge me I made sure I did the judging so harshly that theirs wouldn't compare. I considered placing my baby for adoption while I was pregnant. I felt so loathsome, I thought I had no business being pregnant and was grasping at straws trying to do the right thing. I then realized that someday I would marry, and I'd want my child back. So I chose to keep him, and I am so glad I did. I named him Aiden, and he was my light.

When Aiden was nine months old, I had been praying for a husband. I wanted someone that could be a father to my children, someone that could help me be blessed with an eternal family. I prayed and the Lord said it would be soon. That is when I met Darby. It was a blind date, and I went home and said I could marry him. Two months later, I did. He adopted my three children after we'd been married a year. However, marriage wasn't the easiest. We had many trials that came our way. Our children were struggling from abuse, and we were both struggling with our own difficult childhoods.

One day, a friend gave me a book to read. In the book it talked about visualization and positive thoughts. It also talked about energy. It was an answer to prayers. It felt so right to me, and I knew I had found the answers I was looking for. It wasn't until a few years later that I actually went to an energy practitioner. I was living in a town which was rather close-minded to holistic healing. I didn't want to offend anyone and wanted to serve and honor God. I found someone who was the same religion as me, and I prayed about it. I went and saw her and sent my husband and children to see her as well. After that I wanted to learn more. I felt the light and my connection to Christ grow. I had always known I was spiritually gifted but didn't pay much attention to it. My session with her helped me realize and recognize my gifts.

My husband and I decided we wanted to move back to southern Utah. We wanted healing and more out of life and we didn't feel where we were living was going to provide that. So we sold our home and left for Southern Utah. That is when the healing really started for us. It was neat to see the changes. I had such a hunger for more, to learn more, to be more. It was as if a part of me, my spiritual self was becoming alive again. The true healing I had prayed for was finally happening. I found an energy healing modality that I felt comfortable with. It was in line with my faith. It was simple and effective and made sense to me. I immediately got to work helping others after I was trained. This was such an empowering time for me and so exciting. I was changing and healing, and my family was to. I felt I was living my purpose in so many ways, bringing others out of darkness into the light.

Energy healing is one of those things that people either love or avoid. The funny thing is we are all energy workers and we all move energy every day. If we go to the dentist and he pulls out a rotten tooth what did he do? He removed toxic debris, energy. Our bodies are made out of energy. The science behind it is easy to find if we open our eyes and look. I believe God loves us enough to give us many amazing things that we can choose from to heal. While some may be more comfortable using prescription meds, others may feel better using essential oils. It is important that we remember though that prayer is always first, and all healing comes through Christ's atonement.

As a mother of seven children, I have had many miracles with my children. A few that stand out are those of my two oldest children. My sweet Echo struggled for a long time with her childhood abuse. When she was 18, she became pregnant. This was a tumultuous time. Her self-worth was low, and the programming that she picked up as a young child being abused was running the show. She wasn't sure she'd even raise the baby, and I was considering raising it. As parents, we can only change ourselves. The greatest gift we can give our children is to be healed. I decided that was what I was going to do. I hired a mentor, I did the work, and I continued helping others on their paths bringing them out of darkness into the light. As my life changed, my daughter watched me, and her life changed. She ended up marrying, and is the most amazing mother to her little girl. She just had another daughter in May June 2016. She is active in her church, just graduated from cosmetology school, and is living a righteous life. I owe so much of this to the Christ-centered energy healing that helped her and me.

My wonderful son Draven had his share of trials. In the midst of it all, he was a very gifted woodworker and for years worked alongside me in a business where I made Waldorf dolls and he made wooden toys. Draven decided to serve a mission for our church. This was an absolute miracle. He had everything ready, and then things changed. He was no longer willing to go. He was suffering greatly and in darkness. It was one of those things where you wonder if your child is going to be okay, or if something will happen to them. I didn't give up hope though. On my wall I had a poster with things on it that I wanted to create in my life. There was a photo of two young men in suits. I'd look at it every night and the Spirit would whisper to me, "Saskia, because of the people you are helping, your son is going to be okay." I fasted, I prayed, I loved him unconditionally. I wrote letters to his higher self (spirit). I wrote in my journal about how well he was doing, I focused on what could be, not what was. One day he came to my house; he'd had a life-changing experience and from that day on, he turned his life around. He spent a year working on himself and preparing to go on a mission. He is in Indiana right now, serving his Father in Heaven and helping others.

I run into people all the time that knew me in my youth, and they are very surprised to see how I have changed and grown. Years ago, someone told my daughter not to turn out like her mom. That is truly how some people viewed me because I had such low self-worth. Recently, I decided to surprise one of my mentors from high school. He had not seen me for 15 years. When he saw me and my success, he told me he always believed in me. He said I had something special about me, I had fire, and he knew I'd make it. And I have; I am happy. I have trials and they are rough sometimes, but I am grateful. I surrender to my Father in Heaven, I praise God. I am changing lives by my example and inspiring others. My life will never be the same because I chose to do something different, I chose another way to change my life. I have seven righteous children, and a husband who has completely changed his life. He suffered from deep depression and self-worth so low he says it was put in the toilet and flushed. And now he is mentoring and teaching people. Miracles can happen, if we only open our minds up enough to believe and receive what God sends us. I was sent to this Earth for an extraordinary life, and so were you.

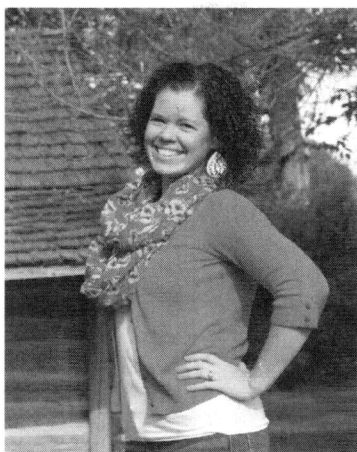

KATIE GARNER

For as long as she can remember, Katie has followed her heart by developing her talent in drawing and painting. She is now an exceptional portrait and mural artist, who is passionate about intentionally creating art that induces positive emotions and conveys spiritual messages. She recently had the opportunity to assist the well-known artist, Linda Christensen, in painting a mural for an LDS temple. She is a Certified Healers Blueprint Practitioner and a mentor. As a loyal wife and devoted mother to five young children, Katie spends her days balancing her family relationships and responsibilities with the many other passions and opportunities the Lord has blessed her with. You can view her portfolio and see what she's creating now, by visiting KatieAGarner.com or by following her on Facebook at facebook.com/ktAgarner.

My name is Katie Garner and I am an energy healer. It has taken me years of studying energy work and assisting in the healing of others to be able to stand up and admit to myself that I have been called to this work. I am finally brave enough to accept that calling and embrace my God-given spiritual gifts. I claim no healing power of my own. On the contrary! Jesus Christ is the source of all healing. I only seek to be a conduit of light, inviting others to tap into the ever-flowing, abundant healing power of the atonement of Christ. I know of no greater work than to assist others in coming to Christ to find healing and hope. Energy work is one tool I use to serve the Lord and assist in His great work.

My energy healing journey started with a struggle to understand personal revelation and discern truth from error. I was feeling strongly drawn to energy work, but I knew nothing about it, and my fear of the unknown scared me. I had a very real, if somewhat irrational fear that if I tried to learn anything about energy work, that I'd find it not in alignment with my fundamental beliefs— that I would somehow be deceived and tricked into a trap of lies that would brainwash me into denying my faith, spiraling downward so far that I'd lose my husband and lead my children down the wrong path, never again to recover, ruining their lives and the lives of their children and their children's children, damning us all to an eternity of heartache and pain, with no chance for redemption! Sigh. You think I'm kidding. I assure you the fear was real. Maybe you can relate.

"There were fears in your hearts, and verily this is the reason that ye did not receive." —Doctrine & Covenants 88:124

So, you could say I was a little resistant to the promptings I was receiving. I thought maybe they weren't promptings from the Holy Ghost at all, but just a strange curiosity I had, or even temptations from the adversary. I brushed off the impressions of the Spirit many times, but the prompting kept coming. In fact, I began feeling not only drawn to it, but practically pushed toward it. Even though I knew very little about energy healing, I began feeling like it was part of my mission in life to be an energy work practitioner and that there were people I could reach just waiting for me to learn how to help them. I was feeling conflicted and unsure. I wanted to jump ahead and know everything before I decided if it was safe to start learning anything at all. Thankfully, God is patient and kind. I had lots of questions. I decided to move forward with faith and trust, taking it one careful step at a time.

"Now, if ye give place, that a seed may be planted in your heart, behold, if it be a true seed, or a good seed, if ye do not cast it out by your unbelief, that ye will resist the Spirit of the Lord, behold, it will begin to swell within your breasts; and when you feel these swelling motions, ye will begin to say within yourselves—It must needs be that this is a good seed, or that the word is good, for it beginneth to enlarge my soul; yea, it beginneth to enlighten my understanding, yea, it beginneth to be delicious to me." –Alma 32:28

A Leap of Faith

Through a series of divine interventions, I learned about an upcoming Christ-centered Energy Healing Conference in Orem during the fall of 2014. I felt encouraged to attend this conference because, after all, it did have "Christ" in the title. I thought I could take a chance on this one, but I'd definitely be on guard! I prayed hard and often, studied my scriptures, and fasted for understanding. I read every scripture I could find about discernment, deception, and how to recognize truth. I pleaded with God to protect me from being deceived. I had enough experience with energy healing to know that it worked, so I felt it had to be either good or evil. I kept asking Him to help me know for sure, and the answer He gave me was, "Keep learning about it and you will know." I wanted nothing more than to follow Him and be loyal to Him. I did everything I knew how to do in order to be prepared to learn by the Spirit. I took comfort in the words of many scriptures and talks at this time, and began having a bit more confidence in my ability to discern truth.

"Striking the balance between trust in the Lord and spiritual self-reliance is a delicate matter, but it is clear that the Lord does not want us

*to be spiritual robots who are afraid to move without first being told
what to do." -Gerald N. Lund, Ensign, July 2004*

One thing was certain. I was either supposed to do energy work, or I wasn't, but I certainly wasn't supposed to sit still and do nothing. It was either a sin to practice energy work, or I was being called to this work and it would be a sin not to follow the guidance of the Spirit . The way to find my answer was to move forward and start learning. So I bought a ticket to the conference.

My First Energy Healing Miracle

A couple of weeks before the conference, my six-year-old son Bryce began having nightmares. He was waking up multiple times every night and coming upstairs to our room in tears. My husband and I would assure him the dream was not real and take him back to bed. An hour or so later, he would return to our room. We prayed together and asked for the nightmares to go away.

I tried applying and diffusing a variety of essential oils to help him relax and sleep. They helped him fall asleep but the nightmares kept returning and he would wake up again. My husband went out of town a few days before the conference and I was left to manage these episodes by myself. I was feeling increasingly more concerned and hopeless about the situation, as day after day continued to pass with no relief. Bryce was beginning to look sickly. His eyes were red with puffy, purple bags under them. He was scared and tired all the time, and I was exhausted too. Three days before the conference, in the middle of the night, while trying to comfort my traumatized son, I plead with God for relief. I admitted that I did not know what to do and that I needed Him to fix this. I had a thought, accompanied by a feeling of peace, that I would find the solution at the conference.

"And I will bring the blind by a way that they knew not; I will lead

them in paths that they have not known: I will make darkness light
before them, and crooked things straight." –Isaiah 42:16

Kimberly Watts was the keynote speaker at the conference. She
was my perfect introduction. She eloquently made it very clear
that she believes all healing comes through Jesus Christ, and there
is no other way to heal. She said that even if a doctor performs
a surgery on a patient, that patient is still being healed through
Jesus Christ. I knew that was truth! She used the analogy of the
sun, the earth, and the moon. She said, "Christ is like the sun, the
people we are helping are the earth, and we are the moon. The
only thing the moon can do is reflect the light of the sun, it has
no light of its own. Any light it shows, is a reflection of the sun."

During our lunch hour, I got a chance to visit Kim's booth and
ask about her program. She began showing me her books and
I suddenly blurted out a question without thinking, almost as if
someone else were speaking through me. I said, "Can you show
me how it works with a live example? My son is having nightmares. How can I help him?" Kim graciously took a few minutes
to work on him, quickly. She didn't have time to explain much
of what she was doing because there was a line of people behind
me, waiting to talk to her. She turned to the scriptures a few times
while muscle testing, which gave me more hope that all this stuff
could be right and good, and she released several things she found.
I didn't understand exactly what she was doing at the time, but I
was filled with peace and overcome with emotion. I stood at her
table and cried as she worked, because I was feeling the Spirit so
strongly. When she finished, she told me there was one last thing
she felt impressed to have me do, as his mother, and his nightmares should be gone for good. She said I needed to go home
and bathe him. That sounded simple enough. Strange, but easy.

I couldn't wait to get home! I rushed out as soon as the conference was over and drove home to my children. I took Bryce

aside and explained to him that I had met a woman who was helping us and that I needed to give him a bath and Jesus would make his nightmares go away. He was excited and, with the faith of a child, never questioned the reality that he would be healed. Before I bathed him, we knelt on the bathroom floor and I prayed for him. He told me afterward that he had smiled through the whole prayer because it made him feel happy. He climbed into the tub and I washed him. As soon as he climbed out of the tub I wrapped him in a towel and we immediately knelt down again and said a prayer of gratitude. I tucked him into bed that night, and for the first time in weeks, he slept through the night. His nightmares never returned. Not once.

It's been over a year since this experience, and Bryce still talks about it. He says to me, "Mommy, remember when you gave me a bath and my nightmares went away? You wouldn't have known how to do that if God didn't show you how. And now I never have nightmares anymore."

Where I Am Now

"If all you know is what you see with your natural eyes and hear with your natural ears, then you will not know much." –David A. Bednar, Ensign, Dec. 2006.

Since this experience, I have sought training from several mentors and teachers and I have witnessed many more miracles. Many experiences have been more miraculous than this. I have discovered and unlocked several of my spiritual gifts that I am still working to develop. I have experienced a massive personal transformation of faith and testimony. I have learned to trust my ability to receive revelation from the Spirit. My perspective and understanding have expanded and brought me more hope and peace than I've ever experienced in my life. The healing power of the atonement has never been so real and present in the here and now for me. I am experiencing a desire to reach out to love and serve others, and I feel a spiritual kinship with all of mankind that is so real I can almost touch it. I feel even more devoted to Jesus Christ and His gospel, and feel so much love and guidance from the Spirit. My confidence before the Lord has massively increased. My prayers are more heartfelt and my scripture study more fervent. I am grateful for the addition energy healing brings to my testimony of Christ. I know now that energy work is only a tool. It is not, of itself, good or evil. The person wielding the tool determines how they will use it. I've discovered that energy is in and through everything, and we are all manipulating energy with our thoughts, words, and actions every day. Educating myself about energy has made me more aware of what I'm doing and how I am influencing the world around me. I am able to be more intentional and have more control over my thoughts, words and actions because I am more aware of the consequences.

Where you search for knowledge is important. Every modality is different. I prayerfully seek inspiration about every class I attend, and every mentor I associate with. I am now a Certified Healers Blueprint Practitioner, trained by Tam Pendleton. I was drawn to her because her program is Christ-centered. I have chosen to put a few practices in place for myself, to protect me from deception and to do my part to be a receptive vessel for the Holy Ghost to guide. I study my scriptures every day and begin and end my days with prayer. I try every day to live like Jesus lived. Every new concept I learn, I weigh and measure against the principles of the gospel that I already know to be true. If it is not in alignment with the gospel of Christ, I do not accept it as truth. I always pray with my clients before every energy clearing session I conduct. I ask God for guidance and protection, and for His will to come forth. My energy releasing medium of choice is prayer. I only use magnets or other releasing tools when inspired to do so. This method has never failed, and it leaves my clients with a clear understanding that it was most definitely not me that healed them, but a higher power, exponentially greater than me.

My prayer for you is that you do not allow fear of the unknown to hold you back. If you are drawn to energy work, trust that you are drawn to it for a reason. Dive in and start learning. Trust God to tell you if this is the right path for you, and trust yourself to discern what the Spirit is saying to you. In all thy ways acknowledge Him and He will direct thy paths.

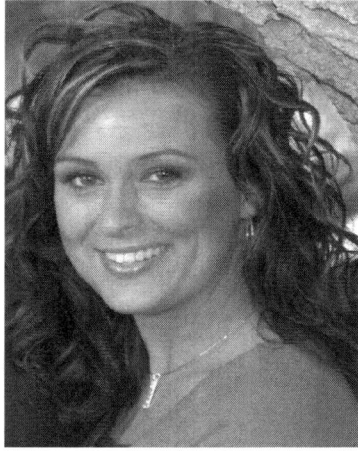

RACHEL NORMAN

Rachel Norman is a Speaker, Mentor & Energy Practitioner as well as a Wife and Mother. She helps couples shift their marriages from surviving into an energy of thriving, as a relationship mentor. She also Founded Walking The Thin Blue Line, which exists to help Law Enforcement Couples and families fortify their relationships. They provide resources for families in Law Enforcement through classes, conferences, & retreats. Rachel's main focus has been empowering couples and families to stay connected and regain closeness while balancing and navigating life. For more information on Rachel and her Programs please visit rachelnorman.com or walkingthethinblueline.com

S piritual gifts. At the core of each of us, we have our own unique set of spiritual gifts. These beautiful and powerful gifts that we have been given have the power to help heal the relationships in our lives and even the generations before and after us. Some of us go about our lives recognizing what our personal gifts are from the time we are very small; others begin to feel a beckoning deep down to come into a deep understanding of their spiritual gifts and who they truly are. For me personally, it was a little bit of both of those situations. From the time I was little I knew that I felt and reacted differently to situations in my life than others around me. I spent a lot of time as I was growing up wondering about how and why I felt the way that I felt. It wasn't until I was older and gained knowledge about spiritual gifts and energy healing that I began to understand my own journey. My journey becoming an energy practitioner and learning to develop my own gifts is what led to the experiences that brought about the story that I want to share with you today.

This story is only able to be told because of the spiritual gifts of some people that I love very deeply as well as the spiritual gifts that I was blessed with in my life. In December 1966, my mother Rani was given up for adoption. She was adopted by two of the most amazing people that I know. My grandparents were beyond excited and overjoyed to welcome my beautiful mother as their daughter. At the time of her adoption, they were not given much information as far as her birth parents were concerned. In fact, it was a closed and sealed adoption. My mother grew up always knowing that she and both of her siblings had been adopted. When she got older, she had tried to find some information on her birth parents, but unfortunately was unable to find anything. As time went on, my mom would mention that she would like to be able to find at least medical information from her biological origin.

On July 29, 2014 I was introduced to someone who became one of my dearest friends and it was through her sharing her spiritual gifts as a healer that this story really began. My sister and I had met Tami at an event at a mutual friend's house. Upon meeting her, my sister and I decided to have a private session with her the following morning. During our session, we were given a message for my mom regarding her biological family. A biological maternal grandmother was felt and was able to confirm several things that had gone on and were presently going on in my mother's life. It could be sensed that she was with us and around us much of the time. She knew and was involved in a lot of the details of our lives. Upon leaving, we immediately called our mom to share with her, what we learned in our session.

In August 2014, my mother became very ill quite suddenly and was put in the hospital for four days. It was during this time that she became more interested in finding medical records from her biological family. I remember her beginning to speak about this a lot more in our conversations after her being released from the hospital.

In January 2015, I awoke one morning feeling very strongly the presence of the maternal grandmother that I knew was connected to my mother's biological line. That first day, I allowed her to stay and be close to me but I was not ready to ask her why she was here or what she needed, though I did pray a lot for her. I awoke the next morning and could still feel her presence along with an intense urgency that she was trying to tell me something. In fact, the urgency was so strong that day, that by that evening I remember sitting on the couch with my husband and asking him if he thought maybe she was around trying to tell me that she had possibly passed away during childbirth with my mother. At the time, I was pregnant with my third child—a baby girl— and really felt like she was trying to tell me something or warn me about something that may be going on with my pregnancy. I awoke on the third morning knowing that I needed to ask her what she needed and follow through with every prompting that I had throughout the day. After I prayed that morning, I sat quietly and took some time to ask her what she needed from me.

I picked up the phone and called my grandma and explained to her that I had this sweet spirit with me and I was in need of her help with some things. My grandma was incredibly open and supportive and allowed me to ask her details she was given upon the adoption of my mom. I shared with her that I was wondering if she had passed during childbirth with my mother at which, point my grandma told me that she knew that my mom's birth mother was alive after giving birth, though I still continued to have a strong sense of urgency regarding the matter. I wrote down everything that she shared with me. I then called my mom and again explained to her what I had been feeling and experiencing in my home. She shared some things with me that she remembered my grandma telling her throughout the years.

Even after speaking with both of them, the feeling urgency would not go away. At this point, I sat at the computer and offered a prayer to be divinely guided and inspired. I also asked this amazing female spirit to help guide me to the information that I needed. I looked up adoption information for Washington state. As I read through the information online, I had found that I was able to print paperwork to send to my mother that she could send in to request a pre-adoption birth certificate. The most incredible part of finding that information was that the state of Washington had actually changed their laws allowing people to request pre-adoption birth certificates on July 30, 2014. This happened to be the exact day that my sister and I had our session with my Tami. I printed off the papers that I found and sent them to my mother. The details that we needed to fill out the forms were very few. I wanted the decision to send in the forms to be fully left to my mother. Upon finding the forms, I could literally feel the love and gratitude of this sweet maternal spirit that had been in our home for the past three days.

I knew that I was divinely guided to do exactly what she had asked me to do. I knew there was a powerful and big reason for her visit. I also knew that several things had been set in motion for my mom to finally get some answers that she'd been searching for in her life regarding where she came from. My mom decided to send the papers. In March 2015, I remember getting a call from her saying that her pre-adoption birth certificate had arrived in the mail and that she had a name and a few other pieces of information about her birth mother. She told me that she never thought she would ever have this information in her life, and that what she had now was more than she had ever expected to receive regarding her adoption. She seemed very content, but mentioned possibly getting on Ancestry.com to see if she could find any other information.

In May 2015, my mother came to be with me and my family for a week during the birth of my daughter. During this time, I thought so much about motherhood, about the deep depths of unconditional love that go along with being a mother. I also still felt that this was not the end of the road for this search. Memorial weekend of 2015, she called to tell me that she had found a picture on Ancestry.com that matched the birth name and birth date for her biological mother. At the moment she saw this picture she had goose bumps and knew that this woman was her biological mother. I think my mom was still trying to decide if she was content with the information that she had or if she was ready to dive head first into vulnerability and reach out.

July 2015, my mom again was getting ready to travel to be there for the birth of my sister's baby. The day before she left to come to Idaho Falls, she told me that she had decided to write a letter to her birth mother and send it before leaving. The night before my mother was getting ready to head back home, she had missed a call on her cell phone. There was a voicemail that had been left from a man named Jack. He confirmed that his wife, the woman my mom believed to be her biological mother indeed was. Her name is Vickey.

The next night on, July 16th, 2016, they were reunited by phone. It was a long-awaited phone call in both of their lives. I could feel the presence that had been with me once more. I also felt several other ancestors in the generational line there with us that day. There were pieces and parts of so many hearts that were healed because of this reunion. My mom and Vickey spent months visiting over the phone getting to know each other better. My mom found out that she also has three more sisters.

On January 29, 2016 my mom, Rani, was able to be reunited with each and every person that she had spent so many years of her life wondering about. This occurred only one year after having my incredible and spiritual experience that helped set us on this path.

I am so thankful that my grandma and grandpa were never anything but fully and completely supportive of how my mom chose to handle the situation, I look up to them so much. My mother and Vickey continue to grow their relationship today. As an Energy Practitioner, I have had the beautiful privilege of seeing so many amazing things. The reason I chose to share this story is because I feel that relationships are one of the biggest reasons that we are here on this Earth. We get to continually work on love and connection with each and every person that we love in this life, while they help to mirror back to us the lessons that our Heavenly Father is asking us to learn. I am deeply passionate about helping others to heal the relationships in their lives and helping them to thrive. More importantly, I feel it is deeply important to share this experience because I know that so many people are coming into a deep awareness of their own spiritual gifts.

They are ready to heed the beckoning from deep within to increase their intuition and their connection to the divine, while developing the gifts that make them each uniquely who they are meant to be. I know that there are some of you out there who are feeling called, who have known that you have always felt different too. I know as we go about increasing our knowledge of spiritual gifts that each piece of the journey is opened up for us at the exact and perfect time. I believe that Rani and Vickey were able to be reunited at the time they were only because that is exactly how it was divinely planned to be. As I look back, there were too many instances that look like "coincidences" that were divinely constructed.

If we are prayerful and ask to know and understand our own gifts, God and our Savior will guide us. They will heal the generational and personal hurts though us. Whatever inspiration you receive, follow through with the promptings that you are given. There were several times throughout this story where I was unsure why things were unfolding the way that they were. I chose to put aside the doubts that I had and instead relied on faith that God knew the bigger picture. I was to simply do what I was prompted to do. If you are being called to do something, to awaken a part of you that is stirring deep inside, you will also be divinely guided to do what has been asked of you. You never know just how deep or how far-lasting the effects of developing these gifts may go. Your gifts can and will have a powerful part to play in helping Christ to heal many lives.

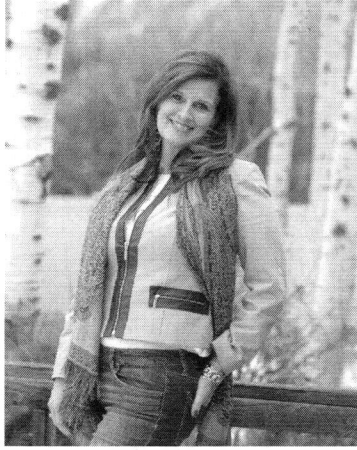

KARYN GRANT

Karyn Grant created "The Healer's Touch Method", LMT, which assists those who are searching for a way to "gracefully transition" through various stages of sadness, sorrow and grief, back into the higher vibrations of love, joy and peace. This Christ-centered approach to wholeness focuses on mending broken hearts and healing wounded spirits with the healing arts of music, massage & aromatherapy.

This deep "Emotional R&R" process goes beyond massage, as it encourages the sub-conscious mind to focus on what is most desirable, while integrating the conscious mind with that intention.

For over a decade, Karyn Grant, LMT, singer/songwriter, has been performing her mission with empathy and enthusiasm. Karyn is the creator of "The Joy Coaching System", which mentors the heart, mind, body and spirit with creativity, empathy and kindness. She is also the mother of "Joy Coaching Nationwide", a group of women who are "Nurturing Heart, Home & Family" using Karyn's methods.

My memories retrace my steps back to the year 2001. I had just graduated from massage school, and had begun praying to know what my next course of study was. *Christ-centered Healing* came the whispered answer to my heartfelt questions. After searching for such a course, I returned to my knees. *Where on earth can I find a course for the healing arts for a Christ-centered Healer?* I petitioned the Lord. *Create one,* came the gentle answer. *Create a course for Christ-centered Healers, using all five senses to awaken the brilliant spirit within.*

I remember the night, my body reeled with exhaustion as I sunk deeply beneath the comforters on my "island bed". I had passed through three more marriages and I was at last, single again and healing from effects of heartbreak number four. In order to do so, I threw myself wholeheartedly into my business of mending broken hearts, as I could totally relate with women who had experienced all kinds of marital mishaps, and who stood in need of their hearts being made whole.

Now, on a Friday night at 7:00 p.m., I felt a wave of sickness passing through my mortal body. *That's unusual,* I thought to myself, *I never get sick.* I muttered a heartfelt prayer for someone to come and minister to me, acknowledging my joy in ministering to others. Two years had passed since opening my new massage business, The Cherishing Place, and I had hardly taken a moment to catch my breath. My CDs The Healer's Touch, Divine Essence and now The Angel Dreams Lullaby Collection had been added to the repertoire of songs and oils completed for processing women and children. It was time to breathe in songs and scents and receive the gift of nurturing with my very own method, created to bless women who stood in need of spiritual rest and emotional rejuvenation.

I had awoken that morning with the very thought, *Do not labor more than you have strength.* Now, I supposed, that this was my body's way of telling me that I needed to rest. I called a friend, who is a massage therapist as well, Kent Smith, and left a message on his voice mail to schedule an overdue appointment. I felt like Martha, finally taking a moment to kneel down like Mary, and choose the good part. Why women feel that they need to press forward and give and give, without taking a single thought for their own needs for nurturing, I do not understand. It is our nature to nurture everyone else. We nurture our baby dolls in our play as little girls. We nurture our pets. We nurture our friends. We nurture our dates. Then we marry, and begin nurturing a husband and children of our own. Even my play as a child was all centered around "Let's play house!". We do what we have always done. But, as Jesus told Martha as he rested in the company of his beloved friend Mary, "It's time for you to rest too, Martha".

As I lay on the massage table, Kent had me breathe in The Healer's Touch oil. I recalled the scripture in Doctrine & Covenants 59 that says, "I have given them the sense of taste and the sense of smell; to gladden the heart and to enliven the soul." Now, as I closed my eyes, I began breathing deeply, allowing all the fatigue to be released from my muscles. I began sinking deeper into a state of tranquility, as though I was being transported with every lengthened breath, into a deeper state of relaxation.

I visualized my worries, my concerns and my troubles all being written on little white Post-it notes, now floating away like little white butterflies, off into a sky filled with light. Deeper and deeper, I felt my mind going into relaxation. I wondered to myself, *Why don't more people allow themselves to receive such peaceful respites along the way of life? This is the best part of the journey,* I thought, as I drifted away into a realm of peace and calm. *These blessed little respites along life's way…*

I recalled the purpose for creating The Healer's Touch Method, combining blessings & blends with compassionate therapeutic touch points. The song, The Healer's Touch was written to recharge the batteries of those who spend their days ministering to others. The lyrics were written to replenish the weary with strength when one is laboring more than we have strength.

Now, Kent was using Flaming Sword. Now, it seemed that my childhood belief that *I am rebellious* came rising to the surface of my thoughts, like dark sludge. Tears began flowing and I whispered quietly, *I never wanted to be rebellious. I wanted to be sweet and loving.* I could hear Kent's voice, speaking to me, like a kind father, words that I had needed to hear for years.

"It's alright, Karyn, breathe out the belief that you are rebellious. Acknowledge it, and let it go." As I inhaled Sweet Surrender oil, I felt the spirit of this self-defense move out of my being like Peter Pan's shadow dancing off with a mind of its own. As the spirit of rebelliousness left my body, having adopted it like an orphaned child at the age of 14, I realized that I had used this as a survival skill to keep my identity intact when I was constantly being told how to think and feel, as a teenager. Somewhere in the process of growing up, I had lost my ability to express my opinions and feelings. But the spirit of rebellion had never completely departed. Another exhale... and I felt my body tingling with an energy that began gathering momentum as it moved from my feet up to my head.

I felt a gentle understanding for the fourteen-year old, realizing that *she* had been doing the best she could in order to survive the misunderstandings, misperceptions and constructive criticism of her well-meaning father. Surely, he had loved her and was only trying to keep her on the straight and narrow. I heard Kent gently whisper, "You don't need this defense anymore, Karyn, you are doing the Lord's work now".

Going through an emotional cleanse is as real as giving birth. I've done both. Now, I could feel the gentle waves of unresolved, unexpressed emotion, ebbing and flowing in soft currents like gentle labor pains, helping to release the pain of what had been left unsaid.

With Sweet Surrender, I was now able to pinpoint and release the need to please others, the fear of giving up my identity if I surrendered my will to others, the feelings of not being good enough, not doing it right enough, and even the reason that had brought me to this table in the first place, the need to run faster than I was able.

The memories surfaced now of when I was a little girl and how often I had felt compared to my older sisters. They were more intellectual, got better grades, were thinner, blonder. In my father's well-meaning attempts to steer me and shape me into who he thought I should be and the direction he thought I should go, I must have gone into over-drive in order to succeed. When I left home, I took over re-parenting myself, placing his values and judgments upon me, first and foremost, right where he left off.

With Magic Kisses, I was able to remember my mother's love and tenderness, like I was discovering a picture in my heart in an old photo album. I was able to feel once more her belief in me and her trust in me, when other well-meaning souls doubted my pure intentions. I was able to mentally cut and paste the picture of her ministering to my little cuts and scrapes in childhood into an image of the Savior ministering to my deeper, hidden wounds.

Breathing in Child-like Faith, I was able to visualize, through the gift of the Holy Ghost, and by my faith in Him, His gift of healing energy spreading through my heart and mind, swiftly sending the melting disappointments of my own defeats and supposed failures in my life.

In the midst of these peaceful thoughts, I heard Kent's whisper, as though he was standing at the end of a long tunnel. His voice sounded so far away.from the place that I had traveled. "It's okay, Karyn, you are doing good things."

Breathing in Scents of Peace oil, I felt my heart moving into a place of greater peace and rest, feeling the assurance that I was truly doing all I could to please my Heavenly Father now, and to bring Him glory. They were like a gentle lullaby to the ears of my spirit. I felt my heart, like a spool of thread wound with too much tension, begin to ease and unwind until my breaths became slower and deeper. I hummed to myself, *There is an hour of peace and rest…unbooned by earthly care…tis when I bring my soul to him and trust his constant care.*

Another soft scent moved my mind back into a distant memory. Perhaps a dream, for me it was a moment of pure truth and tender recollection. It was as though the veil parted for moment to give me comfort from the other side. With this gift of increased insight, I felt joy entering my entire being as I breathed deeply in the soft scent of Pure Love.

The Healer's Touch

In that still moment, while my physical body was in a weakened condition, in my mind's eye, I saw myself sitting on a beautiful green lawn beside the Savior. He was as dear to me, as comfortable to be with, as my very best friend. I felt that I had known Him and loved Him for forever. We were talking together, as easily and as effortlessly as best friends do. There was no feeling of "not being good enough" or "important enough" as I usually felt around other men. In speaking with Him like this, I felt completely safe and secure in His presence. It was a completely familiar feeling to me to be with Him.

All my life, I had always felt inferior to men, but not now. Though I have never had a big brother in this life, I felt very much like His beloved little sister. As I spoke with Him and He with me, I listened intently as He spoke of His dream of going to earth to be a divine healer and to minister to the souls of men, women and children.

As I listened to His heartfelt dream, the feeling that I received from Him was pure excitement, great enthusiasm, and an earnestness to bless His brothers and sisters too. His dream and righteous desires of being a gentle healer was contagious to me! And I thought immediately, *In mortality, sickness is contagious! But in heaven, healing is contagious!*

As I listened to His dream, I felt like Mary of Bethany, sitting at His feet. The thought never crossed my mind that He was in a hurry or that I was taking up too much of His precious time. I felt a spiritual transfusion of pure love and profound energy come upon me. I never once doubted that I could ask anything of Him. I spoke to Him simply, like a little child, saying; *Can I do it too? Can I share your dream with others and become a gentle healer too?* In the very moment that I asked for His blessing upon my kindred desire, He stretched forth His large and beautiful unscarred hand and touched the crown of my head.

As He rested His gentle hand upon me, I felt His dream of becoming a gentle healer spread through my entire being with a sudden flow of energy, eagerness, enthusiasm, a willingness to learn of Him, and an excitement that originated from Him. I suddenly realized from whence the energy had come to accomplish so much in such a little amount of time. This blessing had been pronounced upon my head, in my premortal life, in the very moment I desired and asked for it. The desires in me had been spiritually created before it was created here upon this earth!

Now, I began to be filled with understanding for my life-long dream of touching people's hearts through the gift of song, by sharing the message of the atonement of Jesus Christ. All the puzzle pieces began fitting together in their perfect places. This was His dream before it was my dream! The dream He had shared with me, face to face, heart to heart, in the world before this one!

Suddenly, I knew what I had not known before. The dream I am about is His! I suddenly understood that He is sending and yet will send others into my life who also asked Him, once upon a time, to bless them with healing gifts of the Spirit. I understood that we are not to be competitive with one another, for we have all been given "at least one gift" in addition to the wisdom gained through our individual life's experiences, faith promoting experiences, lessons learned through trial and error, and above all, love for one another.

I realized that the enthusiasm and the excitement I have been given to become a healing instrument in His hands, was indeed a gift from the One who felt it first! *Before this was my dream, it was yours!* I felt myself whispering to him. Before I had the dream to bless broken hearts, He did. I am only an instrument in passing on the contagious feeling I feel from Him!

I know that I do not need to run faster than I am able or to labor more than I have strength. I know that I do not need to carry the burden of healing the whole world upon my shoulders. He already did that. I am only one. The gift of healing is a contagious joy that is meant to be shared by all. As I lay beneath the green satin eye pillow, I wondered of the millennium. In my mind's eye, I could see that there would be thousands upon thousand, who would be striving together to become like Him, all one in our dream of being gentle healers to the family of man.

I wept a little, as I stirred from my restful recollection on the massage table. Kent removed the satin eye pillow and I realize, as I looked upon his smiling countenance just how precious it is to find those dear brothers whose hearts are pure and good and who are willing to share the pure love of Christ and the gift of faith to be healed with their little sisters. Rising up from the table, it was as though I could hear the voice of my Elder Brother, saying, *Take up thy bed and walk, little sister, now do not run faster than you are able, nor labor more than you have strength. Thy faith hath made thee whole!* and then this added injunction, *Go and do likewise!*

I have gone and done likewise. Since that time in 2001 to 2016, I have been ministering to women, men and children with The Healer's Touch Method. It is the purpose that I pursue with passion, knowing that Christ-centered healing is the only healing that can truly bless heart, mind, body and spirit in a way that is lasting and complete; as it gives all the glory to God.

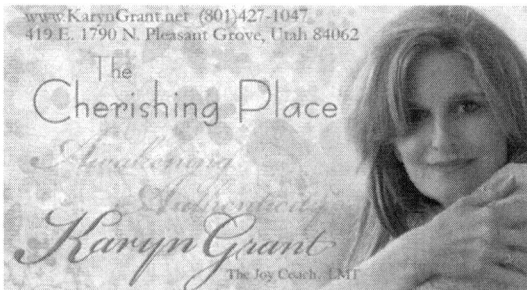

www.KarynGrant.net (801)427-1047
419 E. 1790 N. Pleasant Grove, Utah 84062
The Cherishing Place
Awakening
Authenticity
Karyn Grant
The Joy Coach, LMT

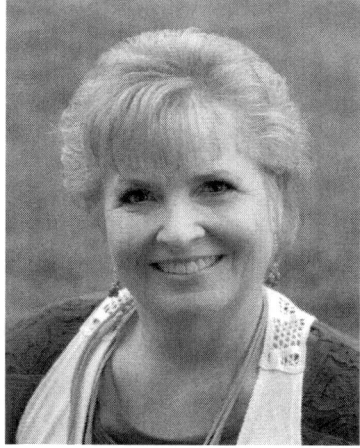

SUSAN TIEDE

Susan is an expert in foot zoning and is dedicated to helping people feel better in every aspect of their lives! She is the owner of Foot Zone Center and has created an amazing and extensive curriculum for teaching the art of foot zoning. Susan has experience in many different educational settings both as a student and as an instructor. It has been her privilege to graduate from three different foot zone training programs whose instructors were all taught by Dr. Ersdal, the founder of foot zoning. Susan also has experience in energy work, mentoring, nutrition, essential oils, herbs and homeopathy. She is motivated by the many miracles she has witnessed in her family and field of work and strives to live a life that is filled with love and gratitude.

My journey as a healer began the day I was born. I was very blessed to be born into a family where my parents had strong testimonies of Jesus Christ. We were taught about Him each day of our lives as we knelt in prayer and relied on the Spirit to guide us and direct us throughout each day.

When asked when I gained my testimony of Jesus Christ, I would have to answer that I believe I have always had a testimony of

Him. I gained that testimony in the pre-existence and brought it with me when I came to earth. My relationship with Him has always been real. He is my Savior, my brother, my friend, and my king. Of course, my understanding and testimony of Jesus Christ has grown as I have journeyed through life and has been the foundation of my work as a foot zone practitioner.

My parents have always been open to alternative ways of healing, which made it very easy for me to have an open mind and believe that a loving God would have many different ways of blessing his children. It was very common in my home to turn to herbs or pioneer methods of healing when one of us was sick or not feeling well. At the same time my parents were very open to the medical world and the blessings that it also offered us in our lives. If they felt that we needed to go see a doctor, they never hesitated to take us to get the help that we needed.

I have always been a very empathetic and sympathetic person towards the needs of others. My tender heart often got me in trouble emotionally. It was very common for me to cry in behalf of my siblings when they got in trouble. I could always see the good in everyone, despite the bad choices they might be making.

I eventually married the love of my life and my very best friend. We have been blessed to have a very happy and wonderful marriage. He is the greatest blessing in my life and my source of strength and greatest support.

After our fourth child Cami was born, I suffered with severe postpartum depression. This was probably the most difficult thing I had experienced up to that point in my life. It didn't make any sense to me that I was feeling the way I did. My life was good and I was grateful that I had a beautiful and healthy baby. All I wanted to do was hold her in my arms and love her but I was so depressed that I couldn't even take care of her. I don't know what I would have done without my angel mother at that time.

She took care of me and she took care of my baby. She bathed her and dressed her and changed her diapers. Then she would hand her to me so that I could hold her with what little strength I had. My mom also took care of my other three children, cooked the meals, cleaned the house and did the laundry for me. I wasn't sure I would survive when she had to go home after being with me and helping me for two weeks.

I eventually saw the light at the end of the tunnel and started feeling better and more like my cheerful self, and then, when Cami was about three months old she passed away of SIDS (Sudden Infant Death Syndrome). This was a very devastating time in my life and I was worried that I would fall back into deep depression. I knew my other children needed their mother and I wanted to be there for them.

Through the love and support and prayers of my family and friends, we were able to get through that difficult time and I actually continued to heal and was able to avoid falling into depression again.

Then about four years later, I was diagnosed with fibromyalgia. I felt like I had the flu all the time. I was in pain and achy every minute of every day. It hurt to move and it was difficult to think clearly. I again suffered with the depression that often comes with the symptoms of fibromyalgia. As difficult as it was to be in pain all the time, it was much easier for me to deal with than the deep dark depression I struggled with.

I searched high and low for the answers I needed to help me overcome this debilitating disease. I turned to nutrition and herbs, and eventually in desperation turned to the medical field and doctors. At one time, I was taking eight different prescription medications. I eventually found some doctors who also practiced alternative healing methods. They were able to help me through some rough spots and give me some physical relief. I was able to get off the medications I was taking, but I still suffered with depression.

I was working with a chiropractor at one time when he suggested that I see an energy healer. I will never forget the day that I was driving to her office to see her when I had this overwhelming feeling that she would be able to help me and that she had the skills to help me overcome the depression I was struggling with. I was very grateful for the confirmation of the spirit on this beforehand or I would have thought her methods of healing to be a little bit strange. But as I sat in her office, I was filled with peace and knew that I had been sent there to receive the healing she had to offer me.

She helped me release a lot of emotional baggage during that first session. She explained to me that I was the type of person who could walk into a room full of people and feel their emotions. I knew this to be true. Although I was far from knowing the details of people's lives and didn't understand what I was feeling, I knew that this happened to me frequently. I would feel heavy, drained and burdened when I was around people, and I didn't know why. She told me that I would unconsciously take others burdens upon myself as it was my nature to want to help others. It was obvious I needed to earn a healthy way to deal with this gift that I had been given. When I left her office, I felt like the weight of the world had been lifted off my shoulders. I don't remember ever feeling more tired than I did when I was driving home that afternoon. I didn't know that sitting in a chair while someone did energy work on me could be so demanding. When I got to my home, I lay down on my couch and crashed. My mom and dad were coming from out of town to visit that day and when they arrived I told my mom that we were going to have pancakes for dinner and she would have to make them. Being a great mom she willingly took on the responsibility. I was able to move from the couch to my bed that night and felt like a new person the next morning. I felt light and happy and more like myself than I had in years.

I continued to work with this energy healer until she felt like she could no longer do anything for me. She suggested that I get my feet zoned and gave me the name of a foot zone practitioner that she felt could help me with the rest of the things that I was struggling with.

My foot zone practitioner, Cara, immediately sensed in my feet the need for me to change my diet in order to clear up a candida problem. She recommended a diet which I started the minute I left her house. I strictly followed this diet over the next six weeks and was able to heal my gut and clear up the overgrowth of candida that was in my system.

I continued to see Cara regularly and was amazed at the results I got from foot zoning. I was grateful for the huge difference it was making in my health. When I watched my diet, managed my stress and got my feet zoned regularly, I no longer suffered from any signs of fibromyalgia or depression.

Cara also taught foot zoning and would occasionally ask me if I would like to learn it. As much as I saw the value in it and loved it for myself, the thought of working with people's feet every day, quite frankly, didn't sound very enticing to me. So I consistently declined her offer, even though she told me she thought I would be really good at it.

At this time in my life, my children were also growing up and leaving home and I had been really praying for answers about what to do with the rest of my life. I had actually been struggling with this for about three years, wondering what it was that the Lord wanted me to do and not really receiving any answers.

One time after Cara finished zoning me, she asked me again if I would like to become a foot zone practitioner. I again told her "no" but as I climbed into my car, I thought maybe I should at least open up my mind to the possibility. I have always been very sensitive to the promptings of the spirit in my life and prayed daily for this gift. It was amazing to me when I opened up my heart the flood of information that came into my mind at that time. I knew that I was supposed to become a foot zone practitioner and that the Lord needed my hands to bless the lives of his children. As I often do when I feel the spirit, I cried all the way home and shared my feelings with my husband. I immediately enrolled in classes and began to learn the art of foot zoning. I knew from the very beginning that this was something my Father in Heaven wanted me to teach and so I put my whole heart and soul into learning this amazing modality. I embraced every opportunity I had to pick up someone's feet and work on them.

I had certified as a foot zone practitioner from two different schools when I felt impressed that I needed to create my own educational materials and start my own training program. I spent the next three and a half years drawing charts and maps of the feet and studying anatomy and physiology and how to incorporate it into foot zoning. My attention to detail and desire for perfection motivated me to keep moving forward. I have written thirteen books on foot zoning and health and wellness. I know that I could never have accomplished what I have without the help of my Savior. Whenever things get hard or confusing I turn to Him for guidance and He always sends me what I need to learn and grow. I love the stories in the scriptures that relate to the washing of feet. There is deep symbolism in these stories for me. I know that all true healing comes through Jesus Christ and that foot zoning is a tool we can use to bless lives. Just as medical doctors use the gifts and talents they have been given to stitch together a wound or heal a broken bone, we can use our talents as energy healers to help others find the healing they are seeking for in their lives. I am so grateful for the advancement in science that is allowing us to measure and see energy, and opening the door for people to be more open to alternative ways of healing.

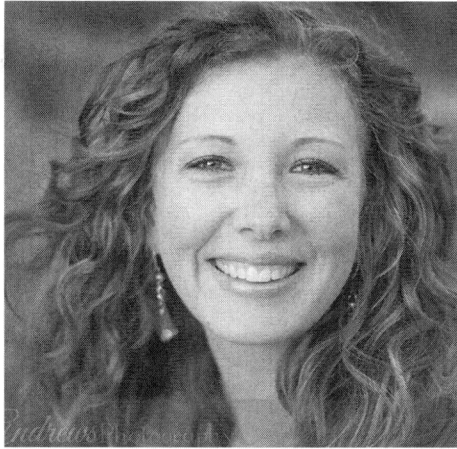

CHANI BIRKNER

Chani Birkner has been helping others to protect themselves energetically for 14 years. She has worked with her parents, Dr. Neil and Cherie Logan, to create new and effective techniques for communication, healing, and self-mastery. She started the website www.cordsoflight.com to help others gain an understanding of principles and techniques that will empower their lives. She has given lectures on topics ranging from energetic shielding to teen communication. She is a multi-passionate person and loves to learn just about anything. She is a second generation homeschooler, and with her husband, Scott Birkner, enjoys raising their five children in Vernal, Utah.

T o explain how I came to know about energy healing and alternative medicine, I really need to tell you of my parents, Neil and Cherie Logan. My parents are people of deep faith in the Savior, and have always done their very best to live by the principles of truth and righteousness. This included admitting when they were wrong, and being humble enough to make right their mistakes.

My father originally set out to pursue accounting as a career, but after failing the final exam (and my father NEVER failed exams,) he decided to take a break and seek guidance from God in his career choice. After prayer and fasting, he was inspired to pursue chiropractic as his profession.

I was very young when my father went into private practice and began to see patients regularly. As he treated them, he found that many of their problems were emotionally based. No matter how much he worked on them, they would only experience temporary relief. He began seeking a way for them to resolve the emotions so they could heal.

My father was introduced to someone who understood *brain language*, and together, my parents learned from her about the principles of working with the subconscious mind. He even sent some of his patients to her. Those patients healed of their emotional trauma, but began to have marital problems. He discovered that the person he was referring his patients to believed that marriage held people back from happiness. He went to my mother and told her that she needed to learn all about *brain language* and energy, and how to apply it in a principle-based way. He knew they had found some truth, and needed to pursue it.

As my parents began using their new understanding of the brain and how to heal emotional trauma, they went to their scriptures even more and began to teach us as children. My father had studied light in the scriptures as a young man, and together as a family we began a lifelong study of the principles of light, what it is, what it does, and how it heals.

I have always had a deep and personal relationship with my Savior, Jesus Christ. As my parents taught us about the scriptures, His life, and His teachings, my understanding of His love for me and for those around me has only deepened over my lifetime. This innate understanding of the divine nature in every person has allowed me to see people as they will be, when the atonement has fully cleansed and purified and exalted them.

Our family scripture growing up was Doctrine and Covenants 88:67.

> *"And if your eye be single to my glory, your whole bodies shall be filled with light, and there shall be no darkness in you; and that body which is filled with light comprehendeth all things."*

As children, we would all gather together before bed and quote that scripture. We would imagine ourselves filling with the Light of God, from our toes all the way up to our minds and then back to God. It allowed us to feel connected to Him. I use this visualization still.

When I was 14, I was given the chance to serve another girl who was close to my age. She had severe OCD and other developmental struggles. She had a baby brother, and her parents asked me to help her watch him for a couple of hours. They wanted her to gradually learn responsibility, but also needed some backup. As I helped her learn the responsibilities of babysitting, my heart reached out to her. The simple things that I did without thought were a struggle for her. She lived in a near constant state of concern and worry about everything from germs to disasters.

Later that night, I struggled to go to sleep. I felt like a huge weight was being pressed against my lungs, and I could barely draw breath. I began panicking, the air was too dirty to give me life, and my mind was racing and teeming with horrible possibilities. I laid in my bed, pleading with myself to calm down, my rational mind pointing out that the air was fine, nothing was on my chest, and I was not thinking clearly. As I reached out in prayer for help, my parents came into the room. I was so faint and struggling to breathe that I couldn't even talk.

Using his skill in muscle testing, my dad quickly discovered that in my attempt to help the sweet girl that day, I had literally taken on her name and identity. My body was trying to be her, and had copied all her anxieties and fears. My mother walked me through giving the identity to the Savior, so that He could take care of it, and then accepting my true identity from Him and restoring it to my body. The instant I did it, I could breathe and talk again! It had been so scary for me, and the relief brought tears of joy to my eyes.

While holding me, my mother explained that it wasn't my role to take my friend's problems and make them mine. That only one person was physically capable of taking upon himself the burdens and sorrows of others, and thus heal them. Whenever we, as mortal beings, try to do the same, it harms us and there is no healing for the other person. She showed me that instead, when my heart is drawn out in compassion for another, that I was to always point the way to the Savior for them to be healed.

In college, I found myself counseling those around me who needed emotional healing. I would call my parents every few days to get further guidance on how to teach the principles I grew up knowing almost instinctively. I finally asked my mother to mentor me, and teach me how to help others heal. Since I was already being sought out for problem-solving and counseling by my peers, I decided I needed to make sure that I had the skills to actually help them.

For the last 14 years, I have worked with my parents helping to heal the lives of others. I have been so incredibly blessed by the understanding of the power of thought, intention, and the ability of the mind and spirit to grasp truth once it is understood. Visualization is a form of intense prayer, and gives direction in a symbolic way to the subconscious mind, giving it instructions in a way it can understand. Using the imagery of light makes something abstract into something tangible, and allows us to trust more of our instinct and intuition.

In 2010, I was pregnant with my third child and I was going through the hardest experience of my life. Scott, my husband, and I were living with his parents in their "new to them" mobile home. We had recently sold our house and had been graciously accepted into their home for the semester while Scott went to school, just a few blocks away. My toddler was sick, and had been since the move a few months earlier. She had what we thought was RSV, but it never got better. We had brought every resource we had to bear on the problem—holistic and medical, and nothing helped. She had a runny nose by day and a cough by night. She wasn't sleeping, and would cry and cry all night long. She also wasn't eating, and she was getting skinnier and paler and had a yellow-tinge to her skin. Our medical doctor had given her one more week to get better, or he was going to have to look into more drastic options.

In a desperate need to get away, we took our little family a few hours away to a friend's house to stay for a three-day weekend. Miraculously, that night she slept all night long and didn't cough once. The next day she started eating, and became ravenous! As we drove back, I just knew we couldn't return to that house. I knew something was killing her there. So, I called my parents, who lived 20 minutes from town, and they took us into their home. We called my sweet mother-in-law and asked her to leave a bowl of water out overnight, to catch whatever was in the air at the house. She readily agreed, being just as concerned as we were about what was causing my daughter to be ill. We took that water into our NAET specialist who uses an energetic technique to resolve allergies, to help discover what was going on. He found that her reaction to the water was the same as the energetic frequency of meth.

We had a company come into the house and test it for meth contamination. It came back at a 6.0! The legal limit at the time was .01 and it was no wonder she hadn't gotten better! My in-laws went to the previous owner, and he agreed to cover the cost of cleaning it up and re-doing the ventilation system. Gratefully, we realized that the house would have killed my daughter, and perhaps the rest of us, and no one would have realized why. My little girl continued to get better and better, her color returned to normal, and she started growing and now slept through the night.

Two years later, though, we discovered that our whole family was suffering from severe heavy metal poisoning, including the baby I had been pregnant with who was now a toddler. Because of the effects of the meth on our systems, our livers had suffered and were unable to do their jobs effectively. So as a family, we went on a whole foods diet that included deep liver cleansing. My little children were having behavioral issues that I knew were tied to the emotions of the event that we had.

There are times when you can be too close to a situation to heal it. This was one of those for me and my parents. My dad was able to work with us on our nutrition and is the one who found the heavy metal poisoning, but we were all too close to the situation to release the emotions involved. The fun part of energy healing is that there are many styles and techniques, and each of them have their specialty. So I reached out to two of my friends to help me figure out and release the negative energy side of our family's struggle.

I believe in throwing everything I have at a problem. I call it *the perfect storm*. That month, we focused entirely on healing—healing our bodies, our minds, our hearts and our energies. It was intense. How grateful I was that I had so many amazing resources and tools to draw on in my hours of need! Our bodies recovered, and the problems that had come up resolved themselves.

It is the worst feeling in the world as a mother to feel lost, without the tools you need to help your children. I realized that even though I had gone through this horrible experience, and it was extremely stressful, I had far more resources and tools to overcome it than most women have.

The techniques and ways of thinking that I grew up with have given me a lot of advantages as a mother. I know how to resolve my children's nightmares within five minutes, which gave us all more sleep. The first thing I check when they seemed irritable and cranky is their energy, and nine times out of ten, filling them with light solves the problem. I know how to connect to them, and help them connect with God. I am able to catch the signs and symptoms of absorbed energy and identity. All of these things are simple, but also have a profound effect. In being so blessed with my life, I am thrilled to now be teaching other mothers those simple tools that they can use in their families and empower them to trust more fully their intuition and connection to the Savior.

Energy or light has been an integral part of my life since I was a little girl. Choosing to do my part, and walk in the Savior's light has been the single most important thing I have done. It is my goal to help every person I can to discover their own connection to Him. We live in a world that has distanced itself so much from the unseen, yet powerfully real world of intuition and light, and so many are unable to trust their own minds and hearts because they were never trained to understand how they work! The term *energy healer* is a new one for me; we always called the techniques we used *brain language* and *emotional release*. If you really understand energy, then you would realize that every kind of healing is energetic at its foundation. I have a deep appreciation and love of all forms of healing. When you do your best to walk hand in hand with the Savior, you will be guided to the healing that you need. That is how you know it all comes from Him.

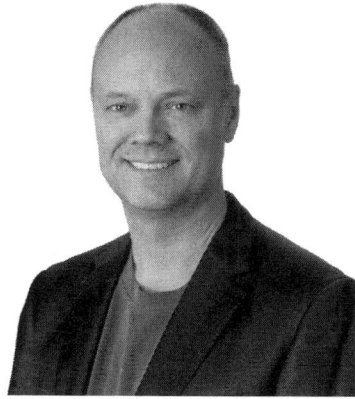

DR. BRADLEY NELSON

Author and international lecturer in bio-energetic medicine and energy psychology, Dr. Brad has successfully used The Emotion Code with thousands of patients around the globe to relieve symptoms and often effect cures in conditions ranging from depression to cancer. His best-selling book, The Emotion Code, offers step-by-step instructions for working with the body's own healing power. Learn more at www.DrBradleyNelson.com and www.TheEmotionCode.com.

My story really began at age seven. I was very ill with the measles, and was confined to bed. My parents had made a makeshift bed for me upstairs in the living room, so that I could be near them. From their whispered conversations about me when they thought I wasn't listening, I knew that they were taking me to the hospital the following morning, or I would be going into something called an "oxygen tent." To my seven-year-old brain, the "tent" part of this plan sounded interesting, but I was really too sick to have enjoyed it.

That night, after everyone else had gone to bed, my parents came into the room. My mother said to my father, "Honey, will you kneel down with me and say a prayer for our boy, that he will be able to get well?" They knelt down by the side of the couch where I was lying, and my father began to pray for me. In the midst of his prayer, I suddenly felt a change take place in my body. This change began at the top of my head and spread through my body to the soles of my feet in the space of about one single second. Within that length of time, I was made completely well. I held my tongue until my father was done praying, which didn't take long. When he finished, I exclaimed, "I'm well! Heavenly father healed me! I'm better!" My parents didn't understand. The reply was, "That's fine, honey. Go back to sleep now. We're going to the hospital in the morning." The next day proved it. I actually was well!

Why do I remember this so well? Well, to go from being very ill one moment to being completely well in the next moment, is something that is entirely unforgettable. That whole experience is etched indelibly into my mind, and if I live to be a million years old, I will never ever forget it. I learned from this experience that there is a higher power, an unseen power that we can draw upon in times of need.

When I was 13 years old, I was diagnosed with kidney disease. At the hospital, the doctors told us that there was no treatment for my condition. They told me to be careful not to run or play too hard, because it could be dangerous. I remember thinking that they didn't really need to tell me that, because just walking would sometimes create pain in my back that would make me feel like I had been stabbed with a knife. Since this disease was potentially fatal, and since there was no medical treatment for it, my parents decided to try an alternative. They took me to see a couple of osteopathic doctors who practiced and lived in a trailer house situated in the middle of a field on the outskirts of town.

Their names were Dr. Alan Bain and Dr. Ida Harmon. "Doc and Ida" started working on me, and within a couple of weeks, I felt much better. The pain that I had been experiencing was much less frequent, and much less severe.

After about a month, I had just about forgotten that I was ever sick. My parents took me back to the clinic, where they ran the tests on me again. The tests were all negative, and as I recall, that was the first time I ever heard the phrase *spontaneous remission*. "Whatever we did must've worked!"—but of course, they hadn't done anything. I knew in my heart that what my "alternative doctors" had done, *had* worked.

I decided then and there that I wanted to be a doctor when I grew up, but not just any kind of doctor.

I wanted to be *that* kind of doctor. If I had to practice in a trailer house in the middle of a muddy field, that was okay with me. Doc and Ida treated people by the busload who'd come to them from all over, even from other states. They were miracle workers, and my life would never be the same after my experience with them.

I remember very distinctly lying on my back on their table during a treatment session and telling Dr. Harmon, "When I grow up, I want to do what you do." She replied, "No, you don't. If you go to school you'll never learn the right way to heal. They'll fill your head so full of dogma and nonsense that you'll never be able to think for yourself again." Maybe it was my age, but for some reason this advice really stayed with me.

As the years went on, my dream of being a healer started to fade a bit. I was introduced to computer programming in college and I loved it. I loved business, and decided that I wouldn't go into the healing arts after all. Instead, I was going to become a businessman.

When I was about six months away from starting the MBA program at Brigham Young University, my wife, Jean, and I went home to Montana for Christmas. As we were sitting with my mother and father in their living room, my father suddenly asked me, "Are you sure you don't want to go to chiropractic school? You've always wanted to do that, and it seems like a really great career." I replied that, "No, I've decided to get my MBA, so I'm really going in a different direction." He said "Well, why don't you think about it one more time?" I told him that I would.

Later that evening, Jean and I drew up a pro and con list. On one side was chiropractic, and on the other side was the MBA and the business world. The list was a little longer on the chiropractic side, but I wasn't convinced. However, I was now not so sure what I really wanted to do. I had thought that my mind was made up, but now I felt like I was being torn between two exciting futures.

When Jean and I got married, we made an agreement that we would never make any momentous or important decision without praying about it to see if it was right. This was definitely one of those momentous decisions. So, that night found me on my knees. I essentially said, "Father in Heaven, if it makes any difference to you, please help me to know what direction to go. I will go either way."

I was awakened in the middle of the night with my mind full of thoughts about healing, and how wonderful it is to be able to serve other people that way. I remember thinking, "Well yes, that's true, but this other direction is good, too...."

I had this experience three times that night. I woke up three times, and each time my mind was full of these "warm fuzzy feelings" about going into the healing arts. Nevertheless, I wasn't convinced. (Do I seem a bit thick-headed to you?)

The next night found me on my knees once again, asking God for guidance. And this was a night that I will never forget. This night, like the night before, I was awakened three times. Each time I was awakened, my mind was filled with the same thoughts as the night before. But somehow these feelings became geometrically stronger and more powerful each time I was awakened.

The third time that I woke up that night, my mind was overflowing with thoughts of service to mankind and to humanity. It's impossible for me to describe what this experience was like. The feelings were absolutely overwhelming, and as my head was filled with thoughts of healing and helping the world, a voice spoke to me.

That voice was crystal clear, and it was as distinct and audible as anything I've ever heard. It said, *This is a sacred calling.*

I've reflected on this experience many times since then. I believe, because the human body is actually a sacred temple for our spirit to inhabit, that any time we are working to help that body function better, we are doing a sacred thing. If we are sewing up an injury, if we are helping someone who is disabled, if we are healing someone who is in need of healing, we are doing a sacred thing.

I ended up going to chiropractic school later that year. It was one of the great experiences of my life, and thanks to my classmates, it was a truly enlightening experience. But even so, I was very much on guard. I remembered Ida's warning to me from many years before, that I would lose the ability to think for myself.

No matter what healing method was taught by my instructors as being the "best way" to fix this or that problem, my attitude was always, "Well, maybe . . . maybe not. Maybe there's a better way to do this. It just hasn't been figured out yet."

By this time, I had become pretty good at computer programming. In fact, I was able to help put myself through chiropractic school by programming the admissions software that our college used. I remember my instructors saying how the brain is the most sophisticated computer in the known universe. I can remember thinking, "Wow, if the brain is really a computer, will we ever have the ability to access the data that must be stored in there, because if we could, it would be amazing!"

I figured that someday, as technology advanced, we might eventually gain this ability. Little did I know how accessing the subconscious database would affect my practice and the rest of my life!

When I went into practice for myself one of the very first patients that I treated was a man who weighed about 300 pounds. He was in tears because he was in so much pain. I remember feeling a sense of panic wondering, "How can I know what this man really needs? What if I don't do the right thing? How can I really help this man to get well as quickly as possible?"

I said a silent prayer to God at that point. "Father in Heaven, you got me into this. You need to help me now, if you will." And He did. Somehow I was able to help that man to get out of pain in short order.

I came to rely on prayer. I prayed all the time for help, although no one knew it. I practiced for 20 years in one form or another, and it was my habit to ask a short, silent prayer of help for each patient that I treated, each time I treated them. I prayed that God would give me the *gift of healing*, one of the spiritual gifts that is spoken of in the Scriptures. I believe I pestered Him for that gift on a daily basis for at least 10 years.

I learned for myself that prayers are answered. My patients got well. There were times, especially during the last years that I was in practice when the patient might present a problem that I didn't know how to deal with, something that I had never seen before, and there were times when, in answer to my silent prayer of help, the information I needed to know would instantly flood into my mind. Sometimes this information was a completely different way of looking at things than I had ever even considered before. I loved my patients. I considered them my good friends. Leaving my practice was one of the hardest things that I ever had to do.

I was a bit like Marcus Welby M.D. If you're old enough to remember, Marcus Welby was a medical doctor, and probably the first doctor show that appeared on TV. During my childhood in the 1960s, it was one of my favorite shows and for some strange reason it made a huge impact on me. Dr. Welby was a general practitioner, a family doctor.

He took care of families, and the show was always interesting because you never knew what was going to happen from one episode to the next. Sometimes, I felt like a family doctor myself. I took care of families, in many cases working with everything from childhood asthma to the problems of old age.

If we can find those imbalances, and fix them, perhaps your symptoms will go away.

As time went on, my patient's problems seemed to increase in complexity as my ability to help them increased. The last 10 years that I spent in practice, I specialized in working with people who were suffering from conditions that were considered incurable by Western medicine. Complex problems like fibromyalgia, chronic fatigue syndrome, lupus, and even cancer.

Consistently I told these patients, "I don't treat diseases. I don't claim to cure diseases. I simply try to find the imbalances that are going on in the body. I believe that the symptoms that you are having are because of imbalances that are going on in your body. If we can find those imbalances, and fix them, perhaps your symptoms will go away." And *go away* they did.

During those years, I saw patients with these difficult problems from all over the US and Canada. The vast majority of them got well, and quite rapidly. I didn't end up helping everyone; my success rate was not 100%, but it was very close to 100%.

Somewhere along the line, I developed this very powerful feeling that people could do a lot to help themselves. I had this deep, driving urge to empower people. I begin teaching seminars to do just that in 1998, and taught as many seminars to as many people as I could around the US and Canada for many years.

I was wearing myself out. I was working in my practice 60 hours a week and then flying off on weekends teaching seminars, and my family was suffering for it.

In 2002, I got a message from "upstairs" that I needed to turn my practice over to someone else, and sell everything I owned.

It had become clear to me that these healing methods that I developed were not just for me or my patients.

These healing methods were for the whole world...including you!

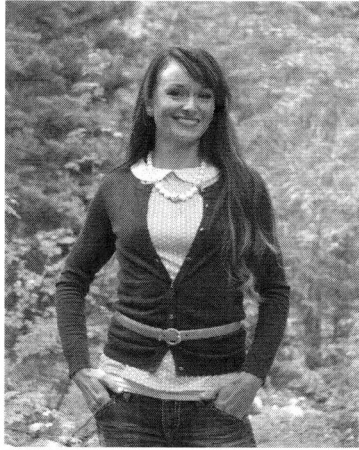

NICOLE STERZER

Nicole was born and grew up in Maryland, then moved to Utah where she met her soulmate Jon. She attended the University of Utah where she earned her bachelor's degree in communications. She and Jon currently live in Utah and have four children.

She loves filling her life with fun-filled fantastic experiences and connections! Nicole is a Christ-centered energy healer.

She is uniquely herself!! Relationships are very important to her. She loves parties, birthdays, color, enthusiasm, burpees, books, swimming and being a sun-shining light with loves and smiles wherever she goes!

Nicole is a food whisperer, author and creator of upcoming classes and cookbook entitled Sanctified & Purified—*clean, pure, delicious, healing eating with love and prayer.*

SanctifiedPurified.blogspot.com

"Give me six hours to chop down a tree, and I will spend the first four hours sharpening the axe." —Abraham Lincoln

We are meant to be *great*! We are meant to be like our Heavenly Parents, therefore we are here to 'sharpen our axe' because greatness is often found in effort and behind the scenes.

We are highly intellectual beings, created after an Eternal Father. Our capacity to grow and learn is infinite. Christ-centered energy healing has allowed me to unlock doors and gifts that have been established in my spiritual being since before I was created.

Growing up I had low self-confidence and esteem. I often felt alone, confused and hurt. I would at times wonder why it was worth living. *I am of no value*, I thought. *I am worthless, ugly, fat . . .* the list continues. I would reach out to those I love and occasionally be told, "Well, I guess you should have never been born." Wow! The sting, the hurt, the anguish and the torment I felt. Thankfully, it was not a constant feeling, but it happened too frequently.

One of the most powerful saving graces of my life during that time was prayer. I wasn't taught spiritual exactness or how or what to say in prayers, I just simply knew that I could pray. What amazed me was that each time I knelt in purposeful prayer to my Heavenly Father, I would be comforted, blessed, calmed and reassured that I had worth. And through all the negative heartache that was swirling around me, I discovered through prayer that I mattered. That I was important. And that I was not alone. The spirit continually worked on me and through Christ's atonement, I was healing. step by step, prayer by prayer, moment by moment. My life overall was not filled with this pain and gloom. I am very blessed. I share this because it is one of my biggest battles I've had to fight. It has also opened me up to tremendous growth.

Fast forward to 2014. My dear beautiful, radiant friend reacted to a prompting for me to go to the Ogden Christ-centered Energy Conference. Months before going to this conference, I was in a fog. I literally felt that I was in this thick sludge and couldn't see, move or have desire to do much of anything. Again, I was confused. Upon going to this conference, things began to change drastically. My mission and purposes in life began to brighten and open up, even though I didn't realize it at the time. I felt peace, joy and my spirit inside me was doing star jumps full of excitement! I needed more. I craved it. It became delicious to me!

Later that year, I attended Kimberly Watts Christ-centered Synergetic Healing Class. I catapulted and I became even more hungry. I realize now, that Christ was pulling me nearer to Him. I was on my path where I needed to go. I wanted more, and so I asked, "How can I achieve?"

Read the scriptures, Study the words of God and attend the Temple often. And so I made it my goal to do that. I was sharpening my axe.

The importance of sharpening an axe before you cut down a tree is that you will have success cutting it down. If we don't put forth the time, effort, ability to prepare and strengthen ourselves, then we will be hacking and whacking at that tree for endless hours while completely exhausting ourselves and not accomplishing our desired goal. However, if we do take the time to sharpen the axe, then we can triple the amount of trees we conquer in less time and with less effort, while enjoying the ride and taking a break to drink a lemonade in between.

All this desire to become,.all this motivation and reaching out is because of Jesus Christ and His infinite atonement! In essence, Christ was changing me and I was allowing it by seeking, pondering, praying and putting forth the effort and desire to become better.

> *"The atonement is, in fact, the most powerful motivational force in the world to be good from day to day" —The Infinite Atonement by Tad R. Callister.*

At the beginning of my marriage, my husband would comple-ment me and I would deny his compliments by brushing them off, or disagreeing with him. It made him unhappy and hurt him that I wouldn't accept his words and believe in myself like he believed in me. At times I would ask, "Why did you marry me?" and his reply was "I know who you can become, and you have a desire and fight to always be better".

> *"And the glory which thou gavest me I have given them; that they may be one, even as we are one. I in them, and thou in me, that they may be made perfect in one and that the world may know that thou hast sent me, and hast loved them, as thou hast loved me." —John 17:22–23.*

Christ was my motivating source and 'fight' in becoming who we are *all meant to be*. We are to be partakers of His gift as we become one with Christ, which enables all His blessings and glory to be ours also. And it all began because God loved us first. He loves us all so much with a perfect love. He is no respecter of persons, He loves you just as much as He loves me. His love is so great that we are perfected as we learn of His love for us and learn who we truly are.

So there is my drive, my motivating force for all good and all good I am and will be! Jesus Christ. He will allow me to grow and to return to Heavenly Father again. Even better, to be *like Him*! He will refine and bless us. God wouldn't refine us, if we weren't worth refining. It is because of Him that I am an energy healer and shine my light because I am reflecting His. It is because of Him that Tammy Ward was inspired to create the Christ-cen-tered Energy Conference. The first one, in which I attended that changed my life astronomically and infinitely for the better.

In the Pail

Two frogs left the safety of their swamp one day and ventured into a nearby farm to explore. Soon they found themselves in a dairy, where they found a large milk pail. Hopping into the pail, they found it was half filled with fresh cream.

The two frogs were absolutely thrilled. They had never tasted anything so delicious! Soon their bellies were full. Feeling sleepy, they decided it was time to leave—and that's when they realized they were in trouble.

They'd had no trouble hopping in. But how were they going to get out? The inside of the pail was too slippery to climb. And because they couldn't reach the bottom and there was nothing for them to step on for traction, hopping to safety was out of the question, too. They were trapped. Frantic, they began thrashing about, their feet scrabbling for a foothold on the elusive, slippery curve of the pail's sides.

Finally one frog cried out, "It's not use. We're doomed!"

"NO" the other frog gasped, "we can't give up. When we were tadpoles, could we have dreamed that someday we would emerge from the water and hop about on land? Swim on, brother, and pray for a miracle!"

But the first frog only eyed his brother sadly. "There are no miracles in the life of a frog," he croaked. "Farewell." And he sank slowly out of sight.

The second frog refused to give up. He continued paddling in the same tiny circle, over and over, hoping against hope for a miracle. An hour later, he was still paddling in his futile little circle. He no longer even knew why. His brother's dying words clutched at his thoughts as fatigue tugged at his tiny muscles. "Was my brother right?" he thought desperately. "Are there no miracles in the life of a frog?" Finally he could swim no more. With a whimper of anguish, he stopped paddling and let go, ready to face his fate....

Yet to his surprise, unlike his brother, the second frog did not sink. In fact, he stayed right where he was, as if suspended in midair. He stretched out a food tentatively—and felt it touch something solid. He heaved a big sigh, said a silent farewell to his poor departed brother frog, then scrambled up onto the top *of the big lump of butter he had just churned, hopped out of the pail and off toward his home in the swamp.*

—*The Slight Edge by Jeff Olson pg. 32–33*

We are the frogs, Christ is the cream, jumping out is our goal. We take leaps of faith into our cream to strengthen us, refine us and eventually after all that we can do and if we just keep swimming, not giving up—we are lifted out because Christ is the changing factor in *all* things. And when we do emerge out of our pot of cream, we can see more clearly at the endless and wonderful horizon! So what can we learn about being a frog?

1. Don't be afraid to jump in! Even as sweet as the cream is, it is still a trial of our faith and takes effort and work to receive more. Everything is always in constant motion and if you are not moving forward, where are we moving?

2. Don't give up! Just keep swimming! After every trial comes great rewards! It may not be when or how we think, but I know they do and *will come!* Have *hope* and *trust* in the Lord and His timing!! *"Blessed is the man (woman) that trusteth in the Lord, and whose hope the Lord is."*—Jeremiah 17:7

3. Have Faith! *"Faith is the substance of things hoped for, the evidence of things not seen."* —Hebrews 11:1 *Isn't that great!* When we have faith, we can have the rewards of heaven and the knowledge of hope in greater things. We can be the frog that knows there is a better way. That is faith and hope!

4. Attitude! An attitude of gratitude will help you see the pot of cream as a stepping stone in your journey and not the end of your journey. Opposition is not fun, but if we embrace an attitude that there is a blessing in all opposition, then it makes swimming in cream for an hour or longer bearable and our gratitude strengthens us along the way. Everything is a blessing, it just depends on how you look at it!

5. Prayer! *"Prayer is the act by which the will of the Father and the will of the child are brought into correspondence with each other. The object of prayer is not to change the will of God, but to secure for ourselves and for others blessings that God is already willing to grant, but that are made conditional on our asking for them. Prayer is a form of work, and is an appointed means for obtaining the highest of all blessings."* —Bible Dictionary. I know miracles happen because of prayer! It is a powerful God-given tool that connects to the Divine. And with God, *nothing is impossible*!! Therefore, miracles can happen for all of us, even frogs.

Through my journey and refining process I have learned these things (and am still learning—isn't it FABULOUSO to learn?!!!!) Through my learning and Christ-centered energy work, I have understood more clearly who I am, why I am here and pieces to my mission in life. I am a divine daughter of God with great purpose! I believe in myself and *all of you* because of our Lord, Savior and Redeemer Jesus Christ paved the way for us! I feel peace instead of sorrow, joy instead of pain and love instead of hate. I *love* who I am and I love people. Each of us has a purpose and reason for being born! And if anyone ever were to tell me again "You should have never been born," I will tell them with complete confidence, "You couldn't be more wrong!!"

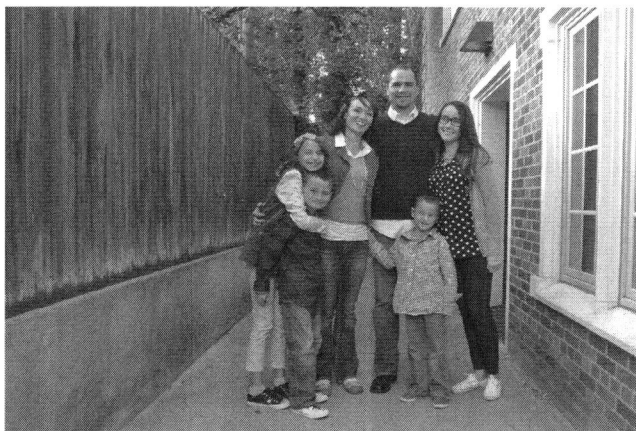

God uses all of His children to bring forth His purposes. We are all a piece to the puzzle, each important; thus together, we are one and complete. Christ is our glue or our 'firm cream' that holds us together. *"Doubt not, Fear not, for the Lord God is with us all! And with God all things are possible"* (Luke 1:37)! I find strength, hope and faith in that statement because it is absolute truth! Lean unto Him and He will make us whole because *we are possible!* LOVES!!!

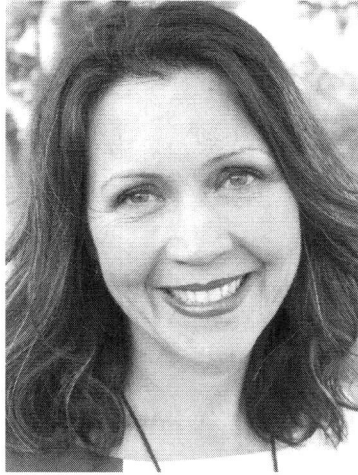

ERICA LAWS

Creator of the Decide 2 Rise NOW series, Erica Laws is a From the Heart mentor, speaker and facilitator of individual life growth. She shares her struggles in life in a transparent and authentic way that touches the hearts of those who cross her path. Her goal in her classes, youth programs, personal mentoring and online classes is to infuse love and light to each human being causing individuals to take personal action to create transformation in their own lives. Erica is a mother of six children with an age difference of 18 years from oldest to youngest. She has worked as a Hospice Nurse and currently holds an active RN license.

Searching is an interesting word. We search for the answer to test questions, we search for the answer to have directions to a destination, we search for many things in life. From the time we are born, we are searching for security and comfort through our mother's care. As we age, we gain an awareness of the need to search for things to help us in whatever task is upon us. When I was five, we lived in the San Francisco Bay area, and I went to a doctor's appointment during the school day. When my mother brought me back to school she let me off and watched me run into my classroom. In those days, (the 70's) nobody signed anyone in or out at the office (at least not at my school). When I ran into the classroom, there was no one there. I was scared and concerned and didn't know where anyone was, so my five-year-old "Erica" instincts said to go home. Home is where security is. Where the answers are. I ran down the sidewalk, for quite a long way, and came to an intersection that I had been told never to cross without an adult. I was told that this intersection was very busy and unsafe. I actually sat down on the curb at that intersection for what seemed like a long time to my five-year-old mind. Eventually, I stood up and bolted across the street running up the block and around the corner to where my home was. My mom looked quite surprised as I came running up scared because of what had happened. I searched for my teacher and classmates and they weren't there. I found out later that they were down the hill at the playground, but, in the moment, I knew getting home was paramount because my mom would have the answers I was searching for.

How does any of this relate to how I have been blessed by Christ-centered energy healing and drawing closer to my Savior? It all relates. Good, righteous mothers, in our lives, come close to the love and comfort the Savior provides. Christ-centered energy healing can help in this area as well. When I was lost as to what to do and came upon an empty classroom, with no humans in sight, the first person I thought to search for was my mother. Even though I had taken quite the trek emotionally and physically! I did whatever it took to search for the one who could provide comfort, guidance and healing.

Everything we search for in life, big or small, is really a searching for comfort, clarity and purpose. The Savior is the ultimate provider of comfort, clarity and purpose. I have found that He wants us to be His hands, His angels, His healers so that we may learn to be like Him. He wants us to let others help us so they may become like Him as well.

As an infant, I searched for comfort. As a five year-old, I searched for guidance and safety. As a middle schooler who wanted to know more about God and my relationship to Him, I searched by getting involved in many different Christian denominations. As a 20-year-old I prayed about a specific book of scripture and a church I was learning about. Because of my searching for an answer, through prayer, I had a direct answer from God, through the Holy Spirit, about who God is, how I am like Him and how I can become like Him.

The warmth of the Spirit permeated every fiber of my being that the words written in the Book of Mormon was truth. It is true scripture from God along with the Bible. As a lifelong learner, I have continued to search to know God's will in my life and do it! Because I have been willing to search to understand and face the depths of depression, suicidal thoughts, addiction, self-hate and self-doubt, I have been guided down a path of healing. I have always strived to increase my testimony of my Savior in my life and have a willingness to find joy, be obedient, repent and become refined. I always am trying to rise above these trials and weaknesses and learn ways to find peace in storm. In the summer of 2015, the Lord made it very apparent that I was to go in a specific direction.

One of my trials and weaknesses is an addiction to food. Why food? Maybe subconsciously, food is *acceptable* vs other addictions. If we are being honest, addiction is addiction. It may show up as alcohol, drugs, pornography, TV, internet misuse, seeking flattery and approval from others or food. Because of this food addiction and unmet emotional turmoil, I was 100 lbs overweight. In 2008, I chose to have gastric bypass surgery. This was a desperate, but not impulsive decision. I knew that initially, I would lose weight, but I also knew that my brain was not being operated on. If I wasn't willing to face the emotional reasons I was eating, then I would gain all the weight back and would be treating the symptom and not the cause. Since 2008 I have worked to be more aware of 'why' I was compulsively overeating, bingeing and turning to food instead of turning to the Lord to overcome my emotional eating issues. I had to face why I was numbing myself with food instead of dealing with the story behind the emotion. Such a simple question, yet eight years later (currently it is 2016), I am still working on those emotional stories, hurts, baggage, lies or whatever you choose to call them. The good news? I have been succeeding by small and simple steps.

So back to summer 2015, I was, for the most part, handling my food addiction, but the bingeing was still creeping in and the dozen glazed donuts eaten over the length of the day was still happening on occasion. I'd chastise myself, turn to the Lord more, exercise and get strict with my nutrition, but the emotion was slow to heal and the cycle would repeat. The emotional issues were healing, but at a snail's pace. I chose to do a 30-day read (it took me 60 days) of a book of scripture that is near and dear to me, The Book of Mormon. The same book I read when I was 20. At the same time, a friend started an online fitness accountability group and I felt it would help me stay on track and stop the bingeing once and for all. Within two days of starting this accountability group and halfway through my scripture challenge, the Lord prompted me to be a health coach. I thought to myself that this was silly. I was currently a stay-at-home mom with a two year-old and several teenagers and they needed me. I was planning on going back to being a hospice nurse when the two-year-old went to kindergarten so why on earth would I be a health coach with a multi-level marketing company? I kind of had some pre-judgments about it all, but the Lord insisted. I did find a simple, clean eating program that helped greatly with the bingeing, but the clincher in long-term change was personal development. I had been more diligent in my prayers and scripture study, so I knew the promptings were from the Lord and I went with it. There was no room for self-doubt. As I said, personal development (which was one of the vital behaviors for being a health coach with this company) changed me in a big way over a period of six months. Not only increased scripture study, but adding personal development reading daily, willing to be vulnerable and sharing my authentic story of gastric bypass and food addiction helped me grow into the person the Lord needed me to be so that, in February 2016, when I was invited to join a one month group mentoring program, I would be at a spiritual and mental level of openness to be presented with the idea that energy healing is real, it is powerful and if it is always Christ-centered, miracles can occur in our lives. I can't even begin to type the tender mercies of the Lord and the miracles that happen daily.

I have met individuals who are Christ-centered and have helped me release and heal emotions and limiting beliefs held since I was a small child. Mental health issues that I have been plagued with since I was at least 13 years old are now understood and honored and confusion lifted. Nothing has been coincidence and the growth that has occurred in my life since summer 2015, and exponentially since February 2016 is substantial.

When I first met with an amazing lady who does emotional release energy work and who had been in my group mentoring class, she guided me through an amazing session of healing. Since then, I have met with her, listened and read about energy healing. I have worked with two personal mentors who have facilitated healing on emotional, physical and spiritual levels. Most importantly, I have stayed diligent in prayer and feasting upon the scriptures to make sure the Lord is my ultimate guide to lead me to those who are centered in Christ.

We have the greatest gift of energy healing or power within us by utilizing prayer and heeding answers from heaven of who we should have in our lives as earthly angels and heavenly angels to facilitate healing. Once we have answers, we have a responsibility to act in faith. With knowledge comes responsibility.

As I stay Christ-centered, I know I will be guided to fulfill my divine purpose to lift others from shame to finding their bright light within. Because of my experiences through Christ-centered energy healing, I am able to help others heal from addictions and emotions weighing them down. Because of my new awareness and joy, I am now able to guide others forward using action steps to reach their full purpose on a divine scale. What joy this is!

Christ has lead me to learn and experience energy healing. This learning, in turn, has lead me to a deeper relationship with Christ, who is my Savior, my Redeemer, my friend and my biggest advocate with the Father. This understanding and clarity has brought into my life the power of God at a higher level. I am surrounded by peace that is beyond earthly. If this is just the beginning of an amazing awareness of Christ-centered energy healing, then I look forward with joyful anticipation to the increased healing power of Christ for my own life, the lives of my posterity and my fellow human beings that I am blessed to have cross my path.

Since I was a young girl attending Presbyterian church camp, one of my all-time favorite scriptures is in Isaiah, *"But they that wait upon the Lord shall renew their strength; they shall mount up with wings as eagles; they shall run, and not be weary; and they shall walk, and not faint"* (Isaiah 40:31).

I am beyond grateful that I am able to be a vessel, a guide, From the Heart Mentor for others to find the healing I desperately sought for so long. Keep searching! All is not lost. There is hope! There is healing!

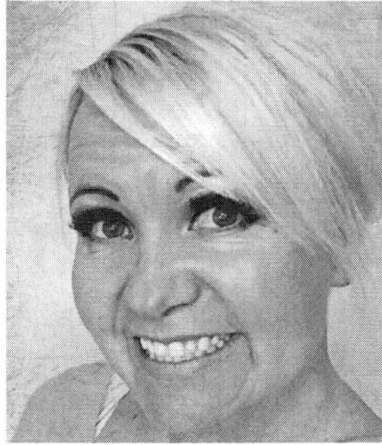

Brenda
Mower-Lindsay

Brenda Mower-Lindsay is the Founder of Spiritually Healed and the owner of Loving Your Life by Brenda. Brenda is a Spiritual Life Coach, Reiki energy healer, and Mentor. She uses a Christ-centered approach to help others grasp the power within as she intuitively leads them through their darkness into their own light. She loves serving our Heavenly Father and her family. She enjoys looking for rainbows after the storms, because she believes that if we can focus on the rainbow we wouldn't mind the storms of life. Her motto is "Always look up and remember who you are"

Growing up in a family of six children, I learned to be a peacemaker. We went to church every Sunday and my favorite lessons were always about when Christ healed the sick and served the poor. He taught me at a young age to serve and to believe in him and to have faith. As a young child, I would live my life in harmony with the Lord, but and as I got older I remember challenging my free agency.

I remember thinking that I just wanted to know what bad was. I just wanted to experience the life of my friends, staying out all night at parties. My life was hard. I lost the spirit and the ancestors that were around me had to leave. I was lost without knowing there was hope in bringing them back. My life began to seem empty and lonely. My father would always say that I needed to change my ways. I was young and wouldn't listen. I didn't want to admit that I was wrong so I would try harder on a road that led to nowhere. I would go out with my friends and stay at their homes.

On my 21st birthday, I was full-term pregnant with my first child. It was then when I fell back on my faith to help me be a mother. I decided at that very moment that I was going to raise my son in righteousness and repent and give him as much stability as I could just like how I was raised. His father left me at seven months along and it was just like the Garth Brooks song, *Unanswered Prayers*.

Years later, I bought some land out in the country and built my son Skyler and I a house. We met our brick mason, fell in love with him and our family was complete. Brett was his name and not being super religious, I fell back into my old ways but with the faith that Brett would change. I was now nine months pregnant again when my true love passed away unexpectedly. I was lost and all alone. Even if I wasn't alone physically, I was mentally somewhere else.

I had a lot of time to think about what I believed in. I would read the scriptures and they would give me peace but it would come and go and my heart would still ache. That is when I started reading only the healings that Christ performed. When I read about Christ raising Lazareth from the dead, it became my favorite story. I was positive that if I had lived in biblical times, I would have searched and found Christ and had enough faith for him to raise my Brett from his passing. And the question filled my mind, *Would you really have enough faith, Brenda?*

It had now been 11 years since Brett's passing. As time went by, the guilt of Brett's death swallowed me up because I didn't call 911 when I first found him. I wasn't alarmed and I always felt it was because I wasn't living righteously. The guilt was like a plague and my faith was weary. Again, I felt lost from my Savior's arms. I was scared and felt in my heart that I was all alone. There were days and nights when I would spend hours on my knees praying to God to take my pain from me. Finally I couldn't stand anymore and fell to my knees and as I cried and sobbed in emotional pain. I begged God, *Why? Why did I have to go through so much when I was so young? I feel so alone.* I heard him say, *My son did not want to either.* It gave me goosebumps and chills and yet I felt the warmth of a bear hug from my Father. My heart had so much warmth burning inside that I immediately asked forgiveness and asked Him to help me always remember this day.

I began wanting to make Him proud of me and I was going to change for good. That very day at work, I was prompted to talk to my long-term patient that I had become extremely close to through the years. She said to me that she felt she needed to tell me about her friend Dusti who was a Reiki healer. She gave me her number and I wrote her a text that very day. I wasn't sure what Reiki even was, but I believe my spirit knew and felt very prompted to find out. We made plans to meet at my dental office in Roy, Utah that following Tuesday.

As the time drew near, it seemed like everything in the world tried to stop us from meeting—phone calls, kids, etc. When she walked through the doors, she looked right in my eyes and said, "Someone doesn't want you to have this session. Lets pray and ask God to be here with us." The Spirit became strong and she proceeded to tell me about what Reiki was. My heart had longed for the healing that was taking place. She explained to me that she knew I had the same gifts of the spirit as she. I knew that night that Christ was there to heal my heart that had once been shattered.

As I thanked Dusti over and over and cried many tears. She told me that it was all from Christ and from his Father, our Heavenly Father.

It was like my prayer to be healed was happening right before my eyes. It was like my life was a puzzle and the missing piece was from the healing that I desperately needed. I knew that night that I could love my life again and be healed. This became one of the most memorable nights of my life! It changed my life in such a way that words can not express. It has now been two-and-a-half years of learning all about how a Christ-centered energy healing can heal lives just like mine. Now it is my mission to help others heal and learn to live with peace and light in there lives too.

I have a stronger testimony of my beliefs and I can now say what I believe to be true. I am a daughter of my Heavenly Father and because I am his daughter, He has blessed me with a gift in helping others through Reiki and the Spirit Code and just listening to the angels all around me. As I continue to learn, I continue to share myself and my knowledge with others. People come seeking me and by the Spirit, I help them. I know that it is Christ that does all healing, I am only a spiritual tool to help Him. My relationship with Christ is the center of my life.

I use Reiki every day in my personal life. I have seen miracles as I am worthy of this gift of energy healing. I honor it and know the importance of why it has come forth at this time on earth. I know that one day, we will have to choose to help others as modern medicine will not be effective. I believe that it was in our blueprint in heaven to come to this earth to help heal and bring people closer to Christ.

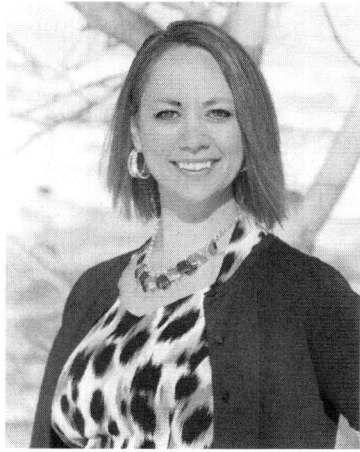

JULIE MAY

Julie has been inspiring youth and adults as a teacher and mentor for over ten years. She is the President and Chief Habit Coach at Excel Your Habits which provides mentoring, coaching, events, and seminars specially designed to help individuals retrain their brain. Her Excellent Habits System is revolutionizing the world of self-help. She is a fiery speaker who excites individuals for change and provides the follow through to make it happen. She is also the producer of the Joyful Living Women's Conference.

For information about Julie's events or the Excellent Habits System, please visit our website at www.excelyourhabits.com.

My husband and I have seven kids between us. Most of them are healthy as a horse. One daughter, however, has been sick since the day she was born. Right after she was born, she had such bad eczema that her entire back looked like one huge scab. There weren't very many positions I could hold her in without her screaming because of the pain she was in. Then there was the asthma, which was the worst case her pulmonary therapist had ever seen. She had been hospitalized for weeks at a time at Primary Children's Medical Center in Salt Lake City.

As she got older, the health problems seemed to get worse, but the doctors had absolutely no idea as to a root cause for any of it. The only thing they could do was to prescribe more and more medication. None of these medications healed my daughter. In fact, the more medications she got, the worse her asthma and eczema got. Each episode seemed to get worse and as she grew accustomed to having steroids in her body, the treatments were less effective.

When she reached about eight years of age, I started looking at alternative treatments for her conditions. About a year prior, she also started having severe stomach pains that would keep her out of school frequently. We started homeschooling her at the time so that we could focus on her health and not have to worry about her missing attendance. My father gave her a priesthood blessing.

I read every book I could get my hands on about how to help heal my daughter. We started learning about foods that would heal her body and how other foods could cause serious damage. I had grown up on the standard American diet of pizza, boxed dinners, and white bread. So this was all new information for me. We changed the foods we fed our family. Out went anything with sugar or white flour. We fed her lots of fruits and vegetables and other whole healing foods. The more healing foods she ate, the less medication she needed. Her stomach pains were coming less and less frequently now.

Our next step in the journey happened when a friend introduced me to essential oils. My sister had used essential oils for her family for a long time, but I knew nothing about them or how they worked. I was having a hard time sleeping at night when I talked to her. So she gave me a trial bottle of lavender and told me to use a couple of drops before bed each night. It worked better than any sleep medication I had ever tried. I had no idea how it worked, I just knew that it did. So I started using other essential oils to help my daughter improve her asthma. When we added the use of essential oils to my daughter's regimen of healing foods, she was able to go several months at a time without using her inhaler when previously she was using it several times every day.

I love learning about how and why things work. I'm not one of those people that is content with just seeing that it works and leaving it at that. I have to know why something works. So I started studying essential oils and learned about how the different vibrations and energies of these substances had healing properties. Every atom in the universe vibrates as do each of the organs in our body. In fact, each of them vibrates at their own frequency. When we find the right essential oil, it can bring those organs into a vibration of healing. One of the great "aha" moments I had while studying essential oils was that as we use these oils, it increases our personal vibration. We also increase our personal vibration as we come closer to God. As our creator, God has the highest frequency of anything ever created. So as we heal our bodies and souls through following God's plan of health, we become more like Him and come to know Him more.

Then I started studying about God's plan for health and we started to rely more on Him and less on the medical establishment. God created a plan for us to have vibrant healthy bodies. He has taught this plan throughout all time. If we read the scriptures and pray to Him, we can learn these things for ourselves. God's plan of health doesn't just include what foods to eat. He teaches us tools for complete health. There are so many laws that we see as spiritual laws which are also temporal laws. There are also temporal laws that affect our spirituality. The more I studied these laws, the more I realized that everything that affects us spiritually affects us physically as well. When He teaches us to forgive our neighbor, it is not just a spiritual law. I found that holding on to anger, blame, or hurt for any length of time can manifest itself as physical pain or ailment later on.

For complete health, we needed to follow all of His commandments. We need to eat the beautiful fruits and vegetables He has created for us, and forgive and love our neighbors and family members. I have known about the atonement from the time I was little. However this was the first time I really started to use it in my every-day life. I didn't just need to forgive people around me, I needed to repent and forgive myself of all of the mistakes I have made throughout my life. As I taught these things to my family, we started to heal more than just physically. Relationships improved and testimonies were strengthened.

A good friend of mine was getting trained as an energy healer when my daughter was about 15 years old. She told me a little bit about how it worked and asked if she could get some of her required training hours by doing some energy sessions with me and my daughter. I was a bit leery at first because I had heard that not everyone who did energy healing was based in the gospel. The modality that she was training in was very Christ-centered and we were still working on some health issues with my daughter (and I was dealing with things at the time as well), so I figured I would give it a try. It seemed to fit with what I was learning about how holding on to negative emotions can cause us to have physical pain. We went in for our first session with her and were amazed at how much she helped both of us and how we felt so much closer to God through the process.

Through Christ-centered energy healing, we were able to heal internal pain and clear emotions that were manifesting as different aches, pain, and ailments in our bodies. As we let go of generations of emotional damage, we both felt lighter, happier, healthier, and another word I like to use is shiny. It comes from the scripture, *"Let your light so shine before men that they may see your good works and glorify your Father which is in heaven"*—Matthew 5:16. As we let Christ's light shine through us by eating pure foods and following God's plan of health and happiness, we become shiny.

We began making appointments with an energy healer each time we started to feel that we were out of sync with something either physically or emotionally. I had started this journey to help heal my daughter. However, I started to realize more and more that I needed healing myself. I had spent so much time and effort on helping her that I had just suppressed anything that I had going on with my own health for years. As I peeled back the layers and started healing myself, I was actually able to help my family more. Many times as moms, we think that we have to sacrifice ourselves in order to serve our family better. In reality, we cannot serve them well if we are not whole ourselves. Thomas S. Monson said, "If you want to give light unto others, you have to glow yourself". I was learning how to glow myself so that I could not only give light unto my children, but to anyone else who was seeking the light of Christ.

Over the last few years, we've been able to heal bodies, cure serious addictions, mend relationships, release emotional baggage, and come closer to Christ through energy healing. I have also studied in the healing arts myself so that I can become a tool to help with my own family's healing. I am so thrilled to be able to share this information so that more people can come closer to Christ and begin their own healing journey. Let's face it. We are all on a journey of healing. Whether our bodies or our souls need healing, we are all broken in one way or another. It is only through Christ that we can become whole. This is the very reason He was sent to earth.

Recently, we went on a car trip for several days. During this car trip, we did not eat the healthy foods that we normally eat at home. Chips, soda, and other junk foods were consumed. We went out to eat a few times and succumbed to breadsticks and other delectable treats at the various restaurants. At the end of the trip, most of us felt physically ill from the change of diet and lack of healthy foods. My eleven-year-old daughter made an interesting observation about this. She asked me if when we got back we could start eating healthy again. I told her that we would and asked if she noticed that her body wasn't feeling as healthy as it usually does, assuming that this was the reason she was asking. She said that her body did feel yucky, but that wasn't the biggest problem. The biggest problem was that she couldn't feel the spirit as well with all the yucky stuff in her body. It was like all of that sugar and junk was blocking her connection with Heavenly Father. Wow. What an amazing observation!

I will be forever grateful for the health problems that led us down this path. Jesus taught us to be grateful in all things, even our trials. Honestly, this took me quite a while to do. I felt like my poor daughter was being picked on with all of her health problems. For a long time, I felt helpless. It wasn't until I turned to the scriptures for help that I truly felt like all the help I needed was available to me. Through our trials, my whole family has learned key tools for really following God's plan for us to have healthy, vibrant bodies and to fully use the atonement in their lives and you can too! He wants to give us the answers we seek if we but turn to Him.

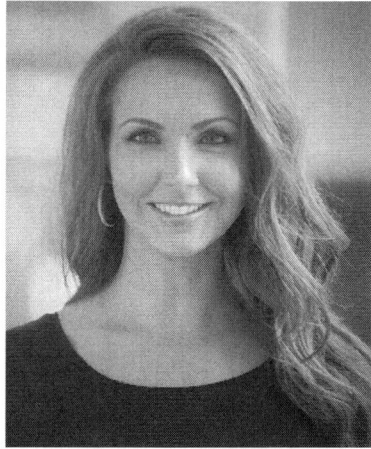

CAROLEE WADDOUPS

Carolee Waddoups is a mother of two beautiful daughters and graduated in 2011 from Utah Valley University as a registered nurse. Carolee is an author, mentor, presenter, and entrepreneur. She loves spending time with her children, being in nature, hiking, running, and progressing in all areas of life. She is passionate about facilitating connections as well as opening hearts and expanding minds in the pursuit of freedom. Her mission in life is to deliver hope and to help others develop meaningful connections to themselves and their higher power, while expanding their vision so they can see their divine potential.

I feel extremely honored to share my experience of Christ-centered energy healing focused on the atonement. I felt an underlying fear from the opposition as I chose this story. There was fear that this particular story didn't belong in this book, wasn't relative, and wouldn't be received well by others. But fear is the adversary's tool and this is the story God wants me to share with you. When I asked for other life events to be brought to mind, I could think of absolutely no other experience. Through the strong urging of the Spirit and after much prayer, I am certain this is "the one."

Please know that the Lord, proper priesthood authorities, and I worked through the process of the atonement together. I asked for and received divine counsel from spirits and people in both worlds so I could understand how the atonement would work specifically for me.

My intention as I share this story is to bring a message of hope so you will know the atonement is real, repentance possible, forgiveness always offered, and unconditional love already yours, given at all times by your loving Heavenly Father.

I was 12. It was the summer before I started 7th grade. My parents had just divorced, my oldest sister had left for college, and my oldest brother was dealing with personal trials and not living at home. My life went from "normal" to chaotic in a matter of months. Then we moved a short distance from our rural home in Corinne, Utah to Brigham City, Utah. I lived with my mom and three other siblings in a small two-bedroom brick apartment in the "bad" part of town. I felt insecure and inadequate with everything in my life.

The girls at church and school seemed fake, mean, and cliquish. My group of friends kept changing and I struggled to feel like I belonged or fit in. I felt incredibly alone. I ached to feel accepted and loved. I felt empty and I was looking for anything to fill that space. I stopped attending church at age 13, and filled the empty space with new cool friends who smoked, drank, and didn't care what anyone else thought. I joined in, believing the lie that this was freedom.

As years passed, I struggled to know who I was. I allowed years and years of physical, mental and sexual abuse to define me. I stood in defiance with my shoulders squared and my chin held high. But just by looking at me, you could not only see the hurt, but feel it. The torture and torment of my soul was tangible. It seeped out of me like a fog, twisting and winding around my body expanding outward to ensnare anyone who dared venture too close. I was cynical, defensive, and wary of anyone who requested anything of me because experience had taught me there would be a high price to pay.

My rebellion and pride hardened my heart and blinded me. I attracted people who preyed on my insecurities. I lost connection to myself, God, and rejected anything good. I was painstakingly proud and pushed people away, yet inside I was screaming for help, for love, for acceptance.

I met Ann when she started working with me as a server in Salt Lake City, Utah. I was hard and cold to new employees, but somehow Ann broke through my walls. She wasn't offended by my cool remarks or the stale smell of cigarette smoke that clung to my clothes. She didn't look at me with judgmental eyes when I changed into *less than modest* outfits after work to go to the club with my friends. She shot straight and surprisingly I really liked her even though I knew she was Mormon.

One night as we were rolling silverware in an empty back room at work, she shot straight like she always did. "Carolee, you have a testimony."

I know there was more to the conversation but I only remember my chest feeling heavy the moment she said those words. I was trying to justify the way I was living, but my spirit recognized truth.

Do you believe in coincidences? I don't. I believe that all things in life are working toward our ultimate good, even the painful experiences. Ann didn't know how much I needed her, but Heavenly Father did. She acted on inspiration, was brave, confident, and faithful. Ann never wavered in her love for me and that changed my life.

Ann was a blessing. A few months before our conversation, I had hit rock bottom. I was in a deep depression filled with self-loathing. I had done something I felt was unforgivable and hated myself for it. These emotions were so strong and volatile that in order to survive, I numbed them. Every night after tucking my two beautiful daughters into bed, I would pour my glass of liquor, sit outside on the concrete steps, staring up to the heavens. I would cry, tears streaming down my face, and beg for forgiveness. I drank to forget and to deaden the fierce pain that exponentially increased when I was alone with my thoughts.

I would remember the appointment, filling out paperwork, the technical tone of staff, and the waiting room. I was all alone... wanting to run... desperately wanting to choose something different but fear strapped me to the chair. I felt there was no other choice, only this. And I remember thinking, *God help me for what I am about to do.*

My thoughts then drifted to the one ultrasound I never saw and the table with the crisp white paper underneath me. The room was cool and I could feel the cold metal stirrups against my feet. I heard the monotone voices telling me about the procedure like it was a common, everyday experience. I stared at the dotted white ceiling tiles, remaining perfectly still while hot tears streamed down my face, filling my ears. There was the sudden, intense pain of an injection. Knowing what it meant, knowing it was just the start and there was no turning back. My entire body trembled as I pleaded with myself, *Keep counting the dots on the tiles, Carolee. Keep counting. It'll be over soon.* The sound of the machine taking the life that was growing inside me hummed in the background. And then it was done. Just like that my baby was gone and I was empty. Hollow. And I wanted to die.

The decision to end the life of my baby wasn't one I came to easily. I wanted to make another choice but was filled with harsh self-criticism and constantly berated myself. *How could you let this happen again?! Didn't you learn your lesson the first two times? Another baby with no father?! What will everyone think? How can you take care of another baby all by yourself?*

I didn't want to be "the screw up" again. I didn't want everyone to know I kept making the same mistakes over and over again, never learning. I didn't want to see the look of disappointment and resignation in their face when I let my entire family down, yet again. The adversary had a firm grip on me and I believed his voice was my own. I fell into his trap of fearing man more than God and believed his lies.

I do not condone taking a life. I am not making excuses or justifications for what I did. I can't bring my baby back or change my past. I share my experience to help others who may be faced with similar circumstances. I made a choice based in fear, believing the lies Satan fed me. The more I believed his lies, the farther I retreated from my loving Heavenly Father.

I went through the motions of life but was being eaten alive with regret, pain, torment, and shame. I knew that I had done something I never thought I would. I knew that in my weakness, I had made the wrong choice. But I couldn't go back. I couldn't undo it, and I didn't know how to stop the pain.

My heart was broken, my spirit contrite. I was reaching out to my Savior but in my sorrow and shame I couldn't hear Him. He knew what I needed, and more importantly, exactly *who* I needed. Meeting Ann was no coincidence; it was a divine gift that saved my life.

I confessed to Ann in a quiet late night conversation. Something inside me knew I could trust her and she held the answers I was seeking. She listened, holding me while I sobbed. She listened to my story, loved me, and saw me the entire time. She whispered the truth of the atonement. She gave me hope to know that I could be forgiven of something I considered unforgivable. Most importantly, she blessed me with the ability to remember what unconditional love feels like.

I released the broken parts of me: the monster and the victim. I actively embraced the light and love the Savior offered me. I started to know who I was. Not who or what everyone else thought I was, but the true me. I saw myself as perfectly imperfect. A finished masterpiece, yet a work in progress at the same time. I began to *see* myself how God sees me.

Repentance and using the gift of the atonement was a process, not something that happened overnight or that I did alone. Ann and her family lived with me for a period of three months, assisting me in separating from old friends, supporting and encouraging me when hard times came. We went to church together and she helped me create positive habits that would sustain me and my children long after she moved out. She was an example, a friend, and in her countenance I saw the Savior.

The atonement was an immersion process. I kept wondering how the atonement could work, but was often reminded to continue taking small steps and stay faithful. I stopped worrying about *how* and began concentrating on *what*. What could I do? What was my next step? Some days my step was to read scriptures, other days to pray, and some days to weep. But for me, true peace came with forgiveness.

"Peace I leave with you, my peace I give unto you; not as the world giveth, give I unto you. Let not your heart be troubled, neither let it be afraid." (John 14:27).

I didn't understand the process I had gone through with the atonement until I read "Power to Become" by David A. Bednar. In his book, I came to learn of the cleansing, redeeming, strengthening, and enabling powers of the atonement which had blessed, changed, and saved my life. You see, once I was able to forgive myself, which was the most difficult part in my journey, I immediately felt the love and peace my Savior had been extending the entire time.

This is my understanding of how the atonement works. When you make a mistake then chose to repent, you are cleansed and redeemed through the atoning power of Jesus Christ. As you continue to make positive changes in your life, both big and small, you are then able to *feel* the cleansing and redeeming powers and access the strengthening and enabling ones. The Savior's love and power add an increase to your own. It is through Him that you grow and progress. When you align yourself with the Savior, you have access to His powers, through the atonement.

I know Heavenly Father knows nothing but unconditional love for you. Your part is to be *willing to receive* His love. As you live and act in faith, you will experience the healing power of the atonement in your daily life. The atonement is real, repentance possible, forgiveness always offered, and unconditional love already yours. I have experienced this and know it to be true. I continually see miracles in my life because of the Savior. Expect to see yours.

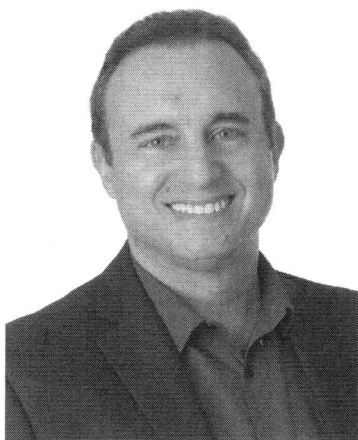

NOAH ST. JOHN

Noah St. John is the founder of SuccessClinic.com, keynote speaker and best-selling author who's famous for inventing Afformations® *and helping busy people achieve personal and financial freedom. His sought-after advice is known as the "secret sauce" in business and personal growth.*

Noah's dynamic and down-to-earth speaking style always gets high marks from audiences. As the leading authority on how to eliminate limiting beliefs, Noah's programs have been called "the only training that FIXES every other training!"

According to Stephen Covey, author of The 7 Habits of Highly Effective People: *"Noah St. John's work is about discovering within ourselves what we should have known all along – we are truly powerful beings with unlimited potential."*

Noah also appears frequently in the news worldwide, including ABC, NBC, CBS, Fox, The Hallmark Channel, National Public Radio, Parade, Woman's Day, Los Angeles Business Journal, The Washington Post, Chicago Sun-Times, Selling Power, Forbes.com, and The Huffington Post.

Get Noah's new book FREE at www.NoahStJohn.com

When I was growing up in Maine, I had to wear leg braces to walk (like Forrest Gump). One day, my pediatrician suggested that I take dance lessons to improve my strength and help me walk without braces. Even though we didn't have the money, my parents somehow found a way to get me into tap class. At first, I was intimidated because I was the weakest, scrawniest kid in the class. But my teacher, a wonderful man named Jon Miele, was patient, kind, and explained every single step to me. He even took the time to write down every step so I could study them after class (yes, I've always been a nerd). That's how I came to take ballet lessons throughout high school. After graduating high school and attending college for one year, I decided to leave college to become a professional ballet dancer...and was broke and miserable the entire time.

A life of dancing is a life of nearly constant pain, both physical and emotional. Sometimes the pain was bad; other times it was really bad. Over time, I noticed that the bad pain was becoming really bad; and the pain that had been really bad was now excruciating. One night on stage during a particularly gorgeous and brutal piece, I was performing a lift when I felt and actually heard something go *pop* in my hip. That was the end of my dance career.

I was 21 years old. I had no money, no connections, no business experience, and no idea what to do with the rest of my life.

I ended up working dozens of "survival" jobs, and was even more miserable than before. I decided to move to Hollywood to become a movie star. A friend from high school let me sleep on his couch until I could find my own place. Having no earthly idea how to get a job as an actor, I went to the library and read books on the subject.

I pounded the pavement, going from one audition to another. But Hollywood was underwhelmed by my performance. Every day was a constant stream of rejection. By now I was living in a tiny apartment, barely making enough to survive, and hoping for my *big break.*

One day in 1991, I auditioned for a traveling musical children's show, and the producer said he loved how I "took over" the audition. Finally! I went home and waited for him to call with my big break.

A few days later, the phone rang. This was it!

"Hello?" I said.

"Thanks, but we've decided to go in another direction." I hung up the phone and decided to kill myself.

No, that's not a simple turn of phrase. When I heard those words of rejection from a total stranger, I decided that I'd had enough of this life. I had been broke my entire life; had never known more than a few fleeting moments of happiness; and spent most of my life angry, lonely, and afraid. So I decided to commit suicide.

Problem: I didn't own a gun. I thought of how I could kill myself without a gun. I remembered hearing how the exhaust from your car engine would kill you in a closed garage. So I decided to do it that way.

Problem: I didn't have a garage, either. In my apartment building, there were only open auto bays, so that wasn't going to work. I decided to find an unlocked garage that I could kill myself in.

Amazingly, I actually found a garage with its door wide open. I could drive in, shut the door behind me, close my eyes ... and that would be that.

Through all of this, ever since the phone call, I was perfectly calm. I wasn't even angry or upset. I remember the moment I decided to kill myself as a crystalline moment of clarity. I had simply accepted that I was going to do it—as simple a decision as going to the grocery store.

But now, staring at the reality of what I was about to do, I paused. *Think about what you're doing,* something said to me. *Are you sure you want to do this?*

And then I saw it: the thing that saved my life.

Parked in the corner of the garage was a child's bicycle. It had a white seat and those white things you hold on to at the ends of the handlebars. It looked just like a bike I'd had when I was a kid.

Wait a minute, I thought. *A family must live here. What are they going to do when they find my dead body in their garage?*

I imagined a woman screaming in shock and terror, a man trying to console her, a child not understanding what happened but knowing something was terribly wrong. I saw my unspeakably selfish act traumatizing this family for the rest of their lives.

And I realized that I couldn't do this to them. Even though I didn't know who they were (and will never know), I realized that what I was about to do wasn't fair to them.

I drove home and got in the shower—perhaps to cleanse my soul as well as my body. As I stood there in the shower, I said, "God, I don't know why you spared my life, but you did. I promise to give the rest of my life to you."

The next day, I walked into a church and devoted my life to serving God . I felt freedom in my soul; I felt born again and renewed in spirit.

I learned how to pray and began meditating and journaling, learning how to quiet my mind and listen to God by following the great example of His son, Christ Jesus. I allowed Christ to come into my heart and accepted Him as my personal Savior. I had a new life and began trusting in God to show me the way.

One day, I was praying when I decided to ask God what He wanted me to do with my life. What happened next was the last thing I expected. I heard a voice say, *Move back to Maine.* The voice came from inside in my head, but the words were as clear as any that had ever been spoken to me.

After I heard the words, *Move back to Maine*, my next thought was, *Are you kidding me?* I hadn't lived in New England for nearly a decade, and the thought of moving back seemed crazy. I decided that it was a silly idea and tried to ignore the voice.

But every time I sat down to pray or meditate, the voice would come back. The more I tried to ignore it, the more I realized that the voice wasn't going away. As I continued to pray about it, it dawned on me that that my time in Los Angeles had served its purpose. I decided to sell my car, my furniture, and most of my belongings, and moved from California back to Maine.

There, I began working with a business mentor who helped me better understand how I could use my talents and skills, I decided to go back to college to finish my degree. In college for the second time, I majored in religious studies and thought I'd end up as a college professor, or even a minister.

And that's how I came to be in my college dorm room on April 24, 1997, experienced *The Shower That Changed Everything*, and discovered Afformations®. You can read more about my discovery in *The Book of Afformations®: Discovering The Miracle of Positive Self-Talk* (Hay House).

On that day, I sat down at my Apple computer and wrote the first Afformations: *Why am I enough? Why am I so happy? and Why am I so blessed to teach and serve others?*

These were thoughts I'd never had before, and the very next thing that popped into my head was: *What am I supposed to do now?* Keep in mind, this was in 1997—years before the advent of blogs and social media; even Google was barely a month old at the time!

I really didn't know what to do with my discovery. I kept trusting in God and taking one step at a time. Then, on October 20th of that same year, I had the second epiphany that changed my life when I discovered *success anorexia*—a condition that causes people to *starve themselves of success*, and leads to behaviors like self-sabotage and what I describe as *driving down the road of life with one foot on the brake.*

That discovery led to the publication of my first book, *Permission to Succeed®*. Shortly thereafter, people began asking me to coach them and help them get their foot off the brake in their lives, careers, and relationships. I coached many clients in my system, and they started getting amazing results—like doubling or tripling their income, getting out of debt, starting new businesses, finding love, healing marriages, even curing insomnia and overcoming addictions!

One month after my 40th birthday, I decided to move to a small town in northeast Ohio. Why? Well, a friend of mine lived there and told me it would be, and I'm quoting here, "fun." Okaaaaaay... Even though I was scared and nervous, I decided to keep my vow to *live by faith and not by sight.*

A short time after I moved to Ohio, my friend introduced me to one of his friends, who in turn introduced me to this gorgeous blonde named Babette. What's amazing about her is that she is just as beautiful on the inside as she is on the outside. I love Babette's values, because she is a believer in Christ and has raised her children that way, too.

Babette and I were married at a perfect ceremony on April 30, 2011—14 years almost to the day after my discovery of

Afformations. At our wedding, in front of our family and friends, I gave her this toast: "Because you loved me for who I am, you made me want to be a better man." And I was crying when I said it!

The years since I turned 40 have been the happiest of my life, because I finally found my Loving Mirror—a person who makes me believe I can do more than I think I can do. I am truly humbled by the opportunity to be an example to my wife and three stepchildren as a faithful, loving husband and father.

Today, our days are filled with family, friends, laughter, and love. I am not only blessed with a world-class support team, I also get to serve amazing clients in over 120 countries and lead life-changing seminars and exclusive mastermind groups for people who come from all over the world to attend our programs.

My books have now been published in a dozen languages, and I'm always grateful when I receive a postcard, letter, or social media post from someone thanking me for something I wrote— whether it's from a person writing from North America, or from a country halfway around the world!

Every night, I still thank God for the gifts of my life—for my beautiful, loving wife and family, our wonderful friends, Mastermind students, and for our thousands and thousands of fantastic clients around the world. I love you all so very much!

I hope my story inspires you to know that, no matter what challenges you're facing, there is a way out—if you forgive the past, step into your best future, and take new actions based on the truth of Who You Really Are. And I would love to help you discover the gifts that God has blessed you with, to empower you to serve and help others on your journey, and to share your message and leave a lasting legacy for your family, your community, and the world.

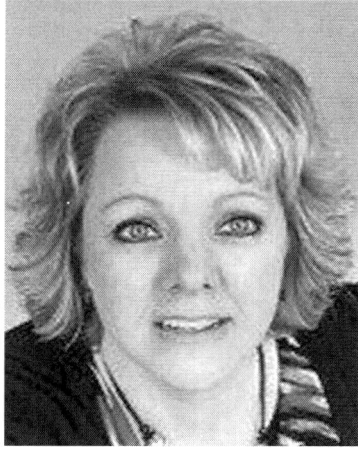

HOLLIE BAXTER

As the owner of a cleaning supply company "Jack Morris Company," Hollie Baxter loves to serve others. She is known as the Ambassador of Integrity and she is passionate about helping others align with who they really are. This love inspired her to continue her education and become certified in Emotional Processing. She graduated from The Institute of Healing Arts and is trained and certified in several alternative healing modalities. She is also the administrator of a social media group "Emotional Health 101." She enjoys teaching others and assisting them on their path to healing through forgiveness. Hollie is a mother of 3 beautiful children and has been happily married for 25 years.

Growing up, I loved school. I loved being with my friends, learning and playing sports at recess. I never missed a day of grade school, and in fact, I received several awards for 100% attendance. School was a place I looked forward to being and felt safe being there. I had several friends that were extra special to me and it wasn't until my adult life that I realized why these kids were so dear to me.

Let me explain. What the kids at school and teachers didn't know about me and my three siblings as well as our mother was that at home, we were growing up with a mental and physically abusive father. I hated being abused although I hated watching my father abuse my mother and siblings even more so. I stayed out of the line of fire the majority of the time. However, that doesn't take away what I witnessed as a young girl throughout my life—things most people think only happen on TV.

Sometime during the summer while we were junior high age, my sister and I walked downtown to the city carnival. On our way home, I felt a sense of urgency to get home. Once we arrived home, I walked in the house, I immediately heard my mother screaming from the other end of the house so I took off running up the long hallway towards my parents' bedroom. Once I turned the corner to their room, I watched my dad beating our mother as she was in fetal position on the floor with her head covered with her arms and hands. I yelled for my dad to stop and when he heard my voice, it was like it took him out of a trance. He stood there and looked and my mother and then at me like he had no idea what happened.

That was the last straw for me. I had watched enough! I personally was tired of being spanked, hit, kicked, and slapped and being whipped with the belt and more so, I was tired of watching my mother and siblings (mainly my brothers) be abused.

Around this same time, my siblings and I made a vow that we would never abuse our children. Never! I remember that vow vividly. All four of us never wanted to be anything like that. I never wanted to get so angry that I hurt others.

After having my own children, I quickly learned that parenting is a bigger challenge than I had imagined. I had two very busy boys that were into everything and tearing stuff apart like normal boys do. I do believe I did a pretty good job parenting them for the most part.

Then I had this experience.

One day, when my boys were little (maybe between ages of 7–11), they were in their bedroom doing something that triggered me to the core. As I approached their bedroom, the door was locked. This increased my anger. I ended up kicking a hole in the bedroom door. When they finally opened the door so that I could see what was going on and see how to discipline them for whatever they were doing, I was so incredibly angry, I knew if I were to lay a hand on them I could possibly kill one of them. At that moment, I remember thinking, *What am I doing? How did I get this angry?* I felt so awful! Later that night as those moments replayed over and over in my mind, I felt numb. How could I allow myself to become what I so desperately did NOT want? I allowed that angry monster to show its ugly head though me towards my precious little boys. How could this be? I made a vow. I promised that I would never do anything like what I watched and encountered growing up. How could this happen? I was better than this! I remember crying and praying and praying and crying, yet I did not feel better. I knew I had to fix this.

Many years went by and I had not learned how to fully control this anger. Once in awhile it would surface, but nothing like that day when I kicked the hole in the door. I had to know where it came from. And most importantly why.

I prayed to understand it and asked what I needed to do to get rid of it and of course, I had repented for that anger over and over.

Fast forward many years.

After my daughter was born, I decided to be a stay-at-home mom. This was harder for me than I thought. I love being around people and when you are a nursing momma you don't get many breaks from the little but very hungry babes. Someone had told me about a place I could take my daughters clothes that she had outgrown and exchange them. That sounded like a great idea as I wasn't working and didn't have the funds coming in that I was used to. The day I felt was a good day to go, I got excited to get out and see something besides my home and the church building that I attended once a week, so I braved the journey alone to Lindon. I went in expecting to find a few cute things for her but when I approached the counter, the lady was very rude and told me that they weren't taking any more clothes that day. I thought and probably said out loud *Are you kidding me?* I have waited weeks to find the right time to come clear over here to do this and now I can't. I was really bothered. I left the store with that angry monster trying to come out as I literally threw the big bag of used clothes in the back of my car and slammed the trunk. I got in my car and felt this strange feeling like this trip is not in vain. *Hum,* I thought, *I am not sure what that meant but okay.* As I continued to back up my car, I literally felt as though someone picked up my car and drove it out of the parking space which was parked facing south and now had me going east into what I thought was a barren parking lot. I was supposed to be headed west to state street, so this was very odd. I followed the prompting and ended up going straight east further into that parking lot. When I got to the end I recognized the name of one business and brushed it off then I pulled into the very end parking space and turned off my car, looked up and saw the sign on the front of the building that said "The Institute of Healing Arts". Wow! Now I was really confused. I got out, walked in and just stood there dumbfounded. I waited for a good solid three to four minutes and no one came. I looked around at the paintings on the wall and the brochures that were lying on the entrance table. It was all interesting. Finally, and older woman with graying hair and a small build came from around the corner and said "Hi, how can I help you?" I remember just staring at her like I had just been dropped onto earth from some planet from outer space and saying "Honestly, I have no idea why I am here". She grabbed my hand kindly and said, "Oh honey, I do!" I just stared at her and then asked questions about the school and what it was. She invited me to come to a free introduction they were doing later that week so I went. I went every month for a while to see if it fit in line with my gospel values and religious beliefs.

I have known for most of my life I had a spiritual gift of knowing things and this was one of those times that I knew that it was good. However, I needed to really know. I prayed diligently for a while to know if that is where I needed to attend and specifically asked Heavenly Father if and when I am to attend this school, would He please have someone call me and tell me that it is time for me to come. Not even a week later after that prayer, I got a phone call from a lady at the school that I had only spoke to once that said those exact words to me. I about fell on the floor. I ended up signing up and taking the year-long course, and graduating with a facilitator's certification in Emotional Release Processing which is considered a secondary education through the state. And guess what happened? I healed! That was the answer to my pleading prayers to heal this anger. It was not only my anger but a generational pattern of anger that stemmed from many generations of abuse. I found the answer!

I finally now more fully understand the true healing power of the atonement of Jesus Christ. I am so grateful for that. It has strengthened my testimony in so many ways too. That year was such a small sacrifice for all of the tools that I now have to help myself, my family and others. The scripture in Matthew 22 that says, *love thy neighbor as thyself* is one reminder that it is required of us to love ourselves. I believe that in order to fully love ourselves, we have to heal from the difficulties from our past and rid those negative beliefs and patterns that do not serve us. Once we do that, we can be more present with our truth. Having the understanding of the Savior's atonement helped me heal; this healing then allows us to further love others more fully.

One thing that I would like the world to know is that we *can* heal from anything the Lord sees fit for us to heal from in this life. It is possible to those that will believe. We are promised that.

The process may be different for others perhaps, but I would like to share what I have learned about healing and that is, that it comes through forgiveness. If someone offends me, hurts me or whatever, we must own our own negative feelings, we must take accountability for them. Those negative feelings do not serve our highest good. They keep us sick and stuck and that keeps our vibration low, none of which is serving us. We must learn to release these in the proper way for true healing.

Here is an example of what I teach others now, many years after healing that anger. I will use my father as an example and walk you through what I have discovered. I would say in prayer "Heavenly Father, forgive me for the anger and hatred that I have in my heart towards my father for all of the abuse I have seen or encountered personally." I would then take a few deep breaths in my nose and out my mouth and then I would ponder or meditate with that for several minutes until I feel a weight lift or a sense of peace.

Sometimes there is a deeper wound that needs to be looked at in further detail in order to get to the root cause in order to fully heal and that would then need to be addressed at that deeper level and that may need to be dealt with through a full emotional release process. However, those tips in and of themselves are powerful. This process is known as neuro-linguistic programming or NLP for short. It walks through what happened, what story was created and what we can do to release it and then create a new story or belief. This is the part I love the most because I get to use my intuition to assist my clients in facilitating their healing.

Through energy work, along with our Heavenly Father's guidance and the Savior's atonement, we can accomplish pretty much anything we desire. Do I still get angry? Yes. Not to that level though as the angry beast is no longer living inside of me and for that I say *Hallelujah*!

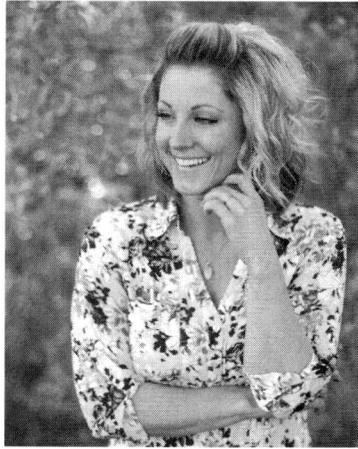

Emma Larsen

Emma Larsen, along with Wendy Mecham is the founder and co-owner of Empower You! Personal Development and Wellness Center. Through many of lifes challenges she was led on a beautiful journey of self discovery. On this journey she discovered a love and gift for healing. Emma has gained a deep understanding and testimony of our Heavenly Fathers unconditional love for each of his children. Through the atonement of Jesus Christ she has found this unconditional love for Her self and all of our fathers creations. It is her life purpose and mission to help others do the same. Emma and her husband Steven reside in Teton, Idaho with their six beautiful children.

Faith

As I begin to share my message of love, hope, faith, and healing through Christ, I feel impressed to pause and offer a prayer for those that are reading these messages at this time. It is through our Lord and Savior Jesus Christ that we find all healing and light. It is through His sacrifice and atonement for all of our Heavenly Father's children that we find hope, clarity, peace, joy, love, and healing. There has never been, nor will there ever be any greater call than that of our Savior's.

I pray now for all of us that we may find this healing and hope in our own hearts and lives and turn unto our Savior and allow ourselves to be cleansed by his great Atonement. I pray that we may all find comfort, peace, and clarity in our own journey of finding faith, hope, and healing. I ask that a blessing be upon all of those reading this book and those sharing their messages that they may be protected and guided on their path to finding that hope, faith, and healing. I pray for these things humbly in the name of our Lord and Savior Jesus Christ, Amen.

In the Beginning

My journey of Christ-centered healing began on the day of my birth. I believe that this healing begins for all of us on the day of our birth by way of the atonement of Jesus Christ.

"For we are his workmanship, created in Christ Jesus unto good works, which God hath before ordained that we should walk in them." –
Ephesians 2:10

I was born in Merced, California in May of 1979. I am the youngest of six children. My parents divorced when I was four years of age. I was raised by an extremely hard working, compassionate and gentle mother. She worked tirelessly to provide for me and my three older siblings still living in the home. Regardless of her many selfless efforts, my family still faced many difficult hardships. Don't we all?

At a very early age, I started experiencing my own hardships outside of the home. Throughout my life I have faced mental, emotional, physical, and sexual abuse. I was also challenged by other worldly obstacles such as addiction, homelessness, two divorces, chronic pain, severe depression, severe anxiety, and many long periods of wanting to take my own life. My journey with most of these obstacles came to an end when I was 26 years old. It began by gaining a testimony of the gospel of Jesus Christ and receiving healing through His great and marvelous atonement.

> *"That through his atonement, and by obedience to the principles of the gospel, mankind might be saved." –D&C 138:4*

Though I found the gospel of Jesus Christ, I still experienced bouts of severe anxiety. I also continued to suffer from chronic pain and migraines. After exhausting my resources with modern medicine, I turned to holistic medicine. It was through the holistic medicine that I was introduced to energy healing for emotional traumas.

Trial of Faith

At the age of 33, while four months pregnant with my sixth child, I started to experience chronic pain again. This pain was physically, mentally and emotionally debilitating. This trial affected me in such a way that I felt a lack of faith in the healing power of the atonement. Just as I started feeling completely alone, I was blessed with the beautiful and priceless gift of friendship. Through my church calling, I became friends with a sweet woman named Joy. Joy told me of her dear friend Leah, a gifted young lady, who practices energy healing. She felt that Leah might be able to help me with my pain. Since I was already familiar with energy healing, I was open to the suggestion.

Several days later, Leah came to visit with me in my home. Immediately, I felt a peaceful and loving energy permeate the room. The pure light she radiated was a great comfort. The Holy Spirit testified to me that she could help me. Through what I would now call spirit to spirit energy healing, she was able to identify the cause of the pain that I carried in my back and right shoulder. As we worked together, she explained to me that much of my pain was generational. This means it was trapped false beliefs, attachments, and emotions passed down from previous generations that were manifesting as physical pain.

To this day, I am not certain which modalities she used to treat me. What I do know is that through a series of muscle testing, and what I would call release and empowerment techniques, she was able to immediately relieve my physical pain. This healing was only possible through the power of God and our faith in the atonement of Jesus Christ. I remained completely pain free for the next five months.

> *"For if there be no faith among the children of men God can do no miracle among them; wherefore, he showed not himself until after their faith." –Ether 12:12*

Healing Through Faith

Two weeks before my due date, I began to experience severe migraines. I was hospitalized one week later due to the severity of my migraines. Upon arrival, they began administering several different medications both orally and through an IV. These medications did little to nothing to alleviate my pain.

The following day, labor was induced and the pain in my head increased. At this time, they feared that I was having a brain aneurysm. My doctor, a man possessing great faith and a testimony of the healing power of the atonement, gave me a priesthood blessing.

> *"In my name they shall heal the sick" –D&C 84:68*

Immediately after the blessing, I was rushed off for a CT scan. Two exciting things happened during the scan. First, it was determined I did not have an aneurysm. Second, my sweet child decided it was time for him to enter this world.

Next thing I knew, the bed I was in was racing through the hall and going down elevators. I was surrounded by my doctor, a nurse and my husband Steven. I am sure it looked just like a scene from a movie. And just like that movie, we made it to the room in the nick of time. In what seemed like less than one minute, our little bundle of joy was there.

Unbeknownst to me at the time, both my newborn son and I would be extending our stay at the hospital. My son refused to eat, so just a few short hours after his arrival, he was admitted to NICU with low blood sugar levels. They attached an IV and feeding tubes to his little body. These treatments were not producing progress towards recovery.

For five days, I had been praying for guidance on what more we could do. It was at this time that I came across my chiropractor walking through the hospital cafeteria and I felt impressed upon to ask him for help and also received a distinct impression to contact Leah.

The next day, our chiropractor returned to the hospital NICU to adjust my child. Immediately after the adjustment my baby was able to void and even eat a little bit. A specialist visited with us after the adjustment and informed us that my son had a weak tongue. They still had no idea how long he would need to remain in the hospital with feeding tubes.

While my son was in the NICU, I was still experiencing my own issues. The doctors kept me at the hospital and proceeded to run diagnostic tests in an attempt to locate the cause of my pain. They continued to pump me full of the oral and IV medications in an effort to ease my discomfort while looking for a solution. These efforts were unsuccessful and I began to experience additional pain in my back.

I contacted Leah on the fifth day post-delivery. She again came to my rescue and was able to assist me through Christ-centered energy healing. Using her spiritual gift of healing with my new faith in the physical healing powers of the atonement, the pain in both my head and back diminished almost instantly.

> *"Now there are diversities of gifts, but the same spirit. And there are differences of administrations, but the same Lord. And there are diversities of operations, but it is the same God which worketh all in all." –1 Corinthians 12:4–6*

She explained to me that I had a nerve in my back that was being adversely affected and she felt that if I would visit my chiropractor as soon as I was discharged, the rest of my pain would go away. At that time we thought the back pain had been caused by the epidural received during labor. Since then, a small hole in my spine has been discovered where the nerves are exposed and are at times agitated. The following morning, I was released from the hospital. I went to the chiropractor as advised and was adjusted. The rest of my pain did go away.

A Miracle Through Christ

Later that evening, Leah met me at the hospital to visit my son in the NICU. After spending some time in his presence, she explained to me that his spirit was not fully present with his body. She explained that my son felt unwanted due to emotional distress experienced during the pregnancy. Leah walked me through the process of spiritually reviewing my pregnancy which allowed me to identify possible upsetting situations and recreate those experiences with positive feelings of love, comfort, peace, and joy. She asked my husband and I to go home that night and imagine our son there with us, coming together as a family, and expressing feelings of love for each other.

Alone in our room we sat as husband and wife while imagining the presence of our son. As we expressed our feelings of love for one another and our child, we felt the flood of the Holy Spirit wash over us. The Spirit testified to us of love that our Heavenly Father and Jesus Christ have for us and that through this experience, our child would be healed.

My husband and I arrived at the hospital early that next morning to find that during the night, my son had started drinking from a bottle as if he had been doing it the whole time. While we were there, they removed his IV and feeding tubes. Within hours, he was released to come home. The joy and gratitude that I felt for this miracle is indescribable. This experience awakened me spiritually. The Holy Spirit testified to me that we truly are spiritual beings of light. I was blessed with a sure knowledge that if I were to develop the gifts that my Heavenly Father gave me, I would be able to help others receive healing. This knowledge instilled within me a great desire to seek my own gift of healing.

"And all these gifts come from God, for the benefit of the children of God. He that asketh in the Spirit asketh according to the will of God; Wherefore it is done even as he asketh." –D&C 46:26,30

Developing my Gifts

Over the next year through studying gifts of the spirit, I discovered that I possess the gift of empathy. This gift allows me the ability to feel what other people are experiencing physically, mentally, and emotionally. This gift is amazing and I am extremely grateful to have been blessed with it. However, in the beginning I found it to be very overwhelming. This led me to seek further understanding of this gift. It was important to learn ways of protecting myself and filtering which experiences I receive. Once I learned this, I discovered that most of my previous anxiety, depression and physical pain had not been my own.

I was able to use my gift of empathy to help others understand what was happening within them emotionally, physically and spiritually. I was also able to help them alleviate some of their pain, with the guidance and power of God. I knew Heavenly Father had a more specific plan for my gifts. So after learning how to manage and use this gift of empathy, I sought His council and guidance on how to proceed. I asked Him what He would have me do with this gift. How could I be an instrument in his hands? What should I do to help bless the lives of others?

"For behold again I say unto you that if ye will enter in by the way and receive the Holy Ghost it will show unto you all things that ye should do." –2 Nephi 32:5

Answering the Call

Through much prayer and meditation, I was led to the healing art of Reiki. At that time, I did not know what Reiki was. After a little research, I discovered that it was energy healing through the laying on of hands. I immediately started seeking a teacher, known as a Reiki master.

It was very important to me to find the right Reiki master. I was seeking confirmation from the Holy Spirit that the Reiki master I learned from was doing the Lord's work. I wanted to be absolutely sure that my teacher was aligned with light and truth. So again, I turned to the Lord. It took eight months before I received my confirmation.

In June of 2015, I found Robin Johnson at the Christ-centered Energy Healing Conference in Ogden, UT. One month later, I attended my first Reiki class. On the second day of class I realized that the work I had been performing, along with my gift of empathy, had actually been Reiki. This revelation cemented my belief that energy healing is true and pure when done through the power of God and the atonement of Jesus Christ.

"And again, I say unto you, all things must be done in the name of Christ, whatsoever you do in the Spirit." –D&C 46:31

I have completed my Reiki classes and have become a Usui/Holy Fire Reiki Master. I have also continued in faith to develop many other gifts of the Spirit. My desire has been to use these gifts to bless the lives of others. I have since been blessed to be able to assist others in finding faith, hope, and healing.

It is my testimony that through this desire to serve others and with the direction of the Holy Spirit, we can assist each other in healing physically, mentally, and emotionally through the power of God and the atonement of Jesus Christ. I am grateful for the trials that led me to this knowledge and to have been called to do this great work.

To conclude, I would like to share my favorite scripture.

> *"And if men come unto me I will show unto them their weakness. I give unto men weakness that they may be humble; and my grace is sufficient for all men that humble themselves before me; for if they humble themselves before me and have faith in me, then will I make weak things become strong unto them." —Ether 12:27*

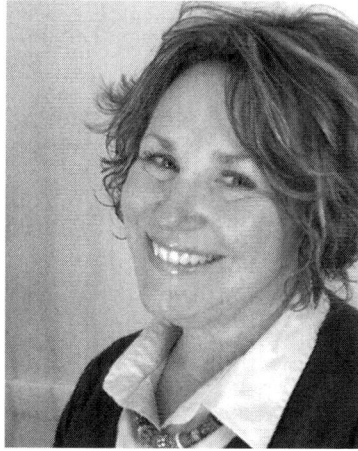

TAM PENDELTON

As the founder of the Healer's Blueprint, *Tam shares a powerful, Christ-centered work that marries intuitive energy medicine/psychology with life skills. Her unique formula for healing uses prayer, energy, and visualization. She teaches others to identify and release patterns of codependency, abuse issues, and limiting programming from the cellular structures of the body. As a skilled mentor and trainer, her Healer's Academy, offers an empowering training/mentoring program for energy practitioners; opening the doors of self-love and empowerment for her students at an international level. She is an LDS wife and the mother of five adorable grown-ups.*

www. TamPendleton.com

When I was 15 years old, a kindly old patriarch laid his hands upon my head and pronounced a blessing of lineage and love. I will never forget it. That sacred moment was the closest thing to heaven I had known on this earth. I was hearing a beautiful story about a strangely familiar version of myself. The words were filled with hope and encouragement from a loving Father who I longed to know. These words were a letter from my long lost heavenly home. It was a glimpse of a dream that I hoped could be real. These words were confirmation that I was valued and cherished as a unique soul with a divine heritage. One peculiar sentence jumped out at me; I was told that my hands would minister to troubled souls and bodies wracked with pain, and that as I met the needs of Heavenly Father's children, He would minister to me in my own need.

I spent years wondering what that meant. At fifteen, in all my wisdom, I figured it must mean that I should be the very best friend I could be. Unfortunately, I came from a dysfunctional, codependent, broken home. I was unaware of my empathetic spiritual gifts. And I was a victim of long-term sexual abuse. So my distorted interpretation of helping other people and being a great friend looked like this: I had to help Jesus by fixing people's pain. In my infinite imperfection, I was such a burden to Jesus Christ that I must save everyone I could, on His behalf. Then I would be helping Jesus, not causing him more pain.

Clearly, I had no comprehension of the Savior's atonement. And I was struggling with a ferocious savior-victim-martyr complex. All of this crazy codependent thinking had me reeling all the time. It was exhausting to live that way.

Against all the odds, I managed to marry Don, a wonderful supportive man. Truly, he was the joyful light in the wilderness. We started a family and enjoyed a good life; it all seemed like a complete miracle to me.

Early in my third pregnancy, we feared a miscarriage. My husband administered a priesthood blessing declaring that the baby would be fine; however, after her birth I would experience a deep and profound depression. And although it would be terrible, I would come forth from that darkness with the strength and understanding to help others overcome darkness in their own lives....It felt like a miracle and a nightmare all at the same time.

Just as promised, I gave birth to a beautiful baby girl and a whopping depression. Don lost his job and went in search of work. Suddenly, I was back in my mother's home, husband and children in tow. Head on, I was facing off with the demons of my childhood. I don't know how my family survived. It was terrible and yet it was a tender mercy. This was my chance to heal the gaping wounds caused by abuse and neglect.

Then along came Lois. She barged into my world with compassion and an understanding of my suffering. Lois dove head first into my deep dark depression. A trained psychotherapist, she was equipped with powerful tools to help me mend. Lois had herself, experienced her own childhood trauma, which led her to become a healer herself, learning to integrate the multiple personalities, or dissociative identities within her brilliantly creative mind. She also introduced me to wild and crazy energy stuff that I had never heard of before, including chakra energy. As Lois described these spinning wheels of energy, I was sure she had lost her mind. After that conversation, I sifted through everything she said, listening for the spirit, making sure her teachings were in sync with my sacred covenants. I had no idea how blessed I was to have her friendship and knowledge.

It took time, and life got better. Soon we welcomed a little son. Without any explanation, Heavenly Father instructed us to move to Utah. It was loud and clear to both of us, so we obeyed immediately. Upon our arrival, we discovered that our dear friend, Tessa had become seriously ill with depression and was hospitalized following after a suicide attempt. Don and I realized it that we had been sent there to care for her during a long recovery. She came home from the hospital to us along with our four young children and our moving mess.

In my humble circumstances and education, I had no previous professional experience that could have prepared me for Tessa. Her mind was shattered by trauma into many dissociative parts, just like Lois. Through her abuse, her trust in God had been destroyed. My hope was to help restore her mind, body and spirit with God and her family. Tessa lived with us for many months at a time, over a period of many years. Some periods of time were profoundly intense and dark. There were nights that as I prayed for her, I feared her suicidal drive would overcome her. I came to realize that each night her room was filled with angelic guardians. I could sleep while they watched.

As I struggled to find the words and the strategies to keep her alive, the Savior showed me that He was the answer. Only his way, only His atonement was powerful enough to repair the breach in her mind. My only responsibility was to show up, listen, love and act on the inspiration given to me. Multiple times I was told, "Just love her better." Eventually Tessa found her way. She has lived a wonderful full life with her family and now her grandchildren.

Later, I would see the sacrifice Tessa made on my on my behalf. She graciously allowed my learning to come at her expense. Though I was trying to lead her to the Savior, it was me that was saved. I found His grace for myself. Her life led me to find the greatest love of my life, as the Savior introduced Himself to me through service. Tessa was lost, so I could be found.

Don and I welcomed another little son in our gray-haired years as forty was closing in on us. I would stay home with him until my turn came to pursue my education in some form of the healing arts. Finally the day, came to follow my dreams for my life. I was told by the spirit to pursue an education as a Licensed Massage Therapist. I was led to study energy healing, energy psychology, life coaching and mentoring. I studied with amazing mentors like Dr. Bradley Nelson, Kirk Duncan, Michael Takatsuno and others. I learned from the best in the world...and yet there was something missing for me. I was not seeing the results I wanted for my clients. Energy work alone was not keeping my clients from creating more negative energy that I was expected to clear away. I was tired of fixing people.

After much soul searching and prayer, (and to my husband's great concern) I closed my Body Code practice. I decided to use life coaching skills to mentor and empower my clients to create more sustainable happiness and positive change. I just didn't know how to blend all of that with my energy skills.

A year later, I sat in a two-day workshop for entrepreneurs, searching for ways to expand my mentoring practice. I had developed a group mentoring/ training helping LDS families to heal. The program was successful and I was determined to take it to the next level. So there I was, longing a little clarity in this little workshop retreat, I wanted to understand why I felt so driven to RUN forward, not very sure where to run! In a quiet moment, as I pondered my next move, a lightning bolt hit me in the head. I was told in a loud clear voice that I was to create my own healing classes for energy workers and healers.

You could have knocked me over with a feather.

It was a ridiculous idea. I mentioned it to a fellow classmate then dumped that idea. My own pride and lack of vision ruled the day.

Two weeks later, in Salt Lake in the middle of my own two-day training filled with men, women and teenagers, the lights went out inside of me. My staff and friends noticed that I was not at my usual energy level. I felt a fog take over my mind. I was fighting for the words to share. Everything went into slow motion.

I became very ill. All the energy systems of my body were shutting down. I had exhausted my adrenals and ignored all the health rules. I set myself up to learn a very big lesson. I was following my purpose to serve others, and help them to heal, but I was no longer on the right path for me. I needed to make a course correction in my life. Though I claimed that I would do as the Lord commanded, when I was told to do shift my direction, I did not obey. I pulled a Jonah. God told me where to go next and instead, I ran the opposite direction. I burned out my body running away from God. There were no whales around to swallow me, so Heavenly Father pulled the plug on my health.

It took a year of rest and reflection to come into submission. Though I completely forgot about the instruction to teach healers, I returned to energy healing. I found my own methods to healing for the subconscious mind in hope of facilitating major change and relief for my clients. I developed a simple mentor/healer program. I wrote it out on post it notes then taped them to my laptop. I got better and better at diving deep into the subconscious mind, and helping others release their pain at a cellular level. I prayed for the keys to opening the mind further for more complete healing.

One Saturday, a dear client/friend invited me have breakfast with him and his wife. He was insistent. He made it clear that his life was forever changed from the work I had done. He wanted me to consider "reproducing myself", by educating others in my techniques and then put it all online. I thought he was crazy. I was a combination of my own healing gifts and every other modality I had ever studied. I had no right to teach other people's materials. *This was impossible!*

Then the big bomb hit. I remembered sitting in a workshop and hearing those words, *You are to create training for other healers.*

I began to process to what my friend was saying to me, "Tam, create a healing program out of all that you have learned then find a way to share it with other healers." For two months, I pondered and prayed for understanding.

One day, as I was working with a dear friend and colleague, a powerful witness washed over me. I saw the Savior laying a crown of confidence upon her head. This was a gift to her as a healer. I also knew that God was ready to answer my prayers. I saw that she was to study with me in depth, and that I was to give her a great gift of knowledge through Heavenly Father. She and I both felt that witness together.

It was a night of intense listening to the spirit. I knew that all I had waited for was coming to me. I prayed to know what to name the "program" that Father in Heaven was about to give me. I called it the *Healer's Blueprint* and secured the domain name. I placed a paper and pencil next to my bed, having NO idea what to do next. The spirit instructed me to go to bed and the information would be given to me in the morning.

A voice woke me at 4 am, calling my name, but only my sleeping husband was in the room with me. I sat up in bed, turned on the light and said, "I am ready". I wrote and drew for a long time. I asked questions. I wrote the responses. It was the greatest outpouring of information I had ever received. After four hours I was told to go to the temple where I would receive more. For three days, the ideas flowed with ease. Two weeks, later the Blueprint chart was complete.

I was clearly instructed that this work was not only for me, but to share with other healers, and that I needed to act quickly. That was in June of 2013.

In August, I was training an academy of 12 talented women on the Healer's Blueprint. It was the easiest, and craziest thing I had ever done. My students knew I had not yet received an explanation or definition for many of the items listed on the Blueprint. It was an adventure in faith and a sequence of miracles that led me to the great Jehovah.

Christ will have His people healed. The Blueprint is for me, another witness of Christ's empowering atonement. The work of Gethsemane is complete. Jesus passed through every ache of our pain and sorrow that night. Now it is up to us to implement that atoning power using our own agency, or forfeit His gift and suffer our wounds and sins alone.

True healers are those who follow the Savior's pattern and direction for healing. In essence, we act as His apprentices. The Master Healer requires that we follow Him in all things. In our efforts to become like Him, we are tutored in His ways to be as He is in all things. Jesus Christ is calling the faithful saints in our day to act on their gifts and witness in His name. Be ready with ears to hear and the heart to answer when He does.

> *"And whatsoever thing is good is just and true; wherefore, nothing that is good denieth Christ, but acknowledgeth that he is." —Moroni 10:6*

You can learn more about the *Healer's Blueprint* at www.TamPendleton.com.

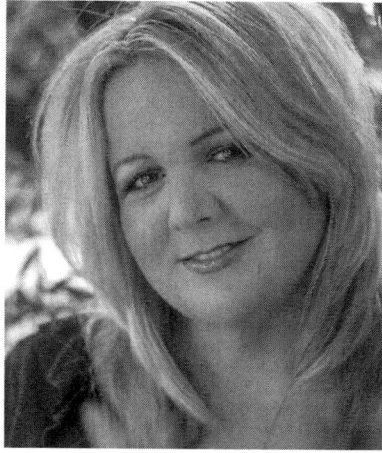

CHRISTI TURLEY DIAMOND

Christi Turley Diamond B.S., M.Ed., is a speaker, author, life coach and intuitive energy healer. She is certified as a Grief & Loss Recovery Specialist and worked for years in a non-profit organization assisting many affected by loss and trauma. She is the co-author of Aroma Heal 1 & 2 and creator of the Aroma Heal certification program. She does individual/group phone sessions with clients all over the world. She has helped hundreds to find healing. Her purpose is to increase light upon the earth as she helps others recognize and increase theirs. You can find her at www.thehealingcoach.com.

When I was two, my grandpa used to call me "big brown eyes". My eyes were large and a dominant feature on my little face. They say the eyes are the mirror to the soul. I have beautiful chocolate brown eyes and if you look long and deeply enough, you might see etchings of pain, but around the edges you will see the hope embedded deep in my soul and the light within that was created from a deep sense of compassion and immeasurable wisdom from life experiences that have shaped me into the giver and healer I am today. My greatest heartaches have become my greatest teachers. My greatest healer has been Jesus Christ. He is where my light shines brightest.

I think back even to a few short years ago and recognize how different my life is today because I was willing to invest in myself and in my own healing. Today I am a completely different person. I think of all the life-changing effects on my own life using energy healing and concepts I now know and I stand in awe. I have experienced my marriage literally transform into what I've always wanted it to be. My relationship with self and my business have been equally transformational. All because I was finally willing to face truth.

As I have participated in healing work through the healing power of Jesus Christ on a regular basis, I have felt lighter, confidence in myself has grown, and so has my belief in myself. I have been able to let go of old patterns and cycles in the past that held me back. I feel joy and such a peace that at times is indescribable. It's a place I never want to leave.

This was not at all where I was 10 years ago. Sometimes our mess becomes our message. My life 10 years ago does not even resemble what it is today. I was experiencing a horrible divorce, became mom and dad 24/7 to three young boys, and found myself homeless, broke and moving to another city to have a roof over our heads. I thought my life was over. Little did I know, it was just beginning. I had lost any belief in myself and I was in a dark place. I felt alone and full of questions. I didn't really know what my purpose was or what I was here to do that was unique to me.

I was a miserable person. I compared myself to everyone and thought life was all about what fate dealt you. I was just existing and trying to be better and yet I complained *a lot*, so I criticized and judged myself and others harshly. I thought that I wasn't deserving of happiness. Betrayal on every level had reared its ugly head. I questioned everything I thought I knew and I doubted myself completely. I lost trust in myself and the walls around me became a fortress of protection.

As I experienced divorce, I became clinically depressed and literally prayed to die! I clearly remember being on me knees, in my closet crying and begging and pleading with the Lord to take me. The heart-wrenching pain was so unbearable that there were days it took my breath away. Everything I believed in was shattered and I felt broken, My heart was crumbling into a million pieces, never to be put back together again. I had three young boys to care for, and I was praying to die! That's how low I felt in the dark place I existed in. I thought my life was over because it didn't go the way I planned it. I had experienced abuse on all levels and I felt I had done everything in my power for life to be different and better. I was a prisoner to my own thoughts and beliefs. I didn't know any different so I was doing the best I could with what I knew. I had no clue as to how stuck I really was.

I pushed through and tried to overcome by immersing myself in self development books to try and fix all my brokenness. I was saying daily affirmations over and over, trying so hard to *convince* myself that I was rich or happy or successful, and honestly, it worked for me…for a little while. I'm not knocking self development at all. I totally believe in it and I still read books daily because I find great value in them and gain much insight, *but* it wasn't until I finally got to the core of healing within that I started getting *huge* results in my life, where I *felt* successful and happy and abundant! There is quite a difference in convincing ourselves, as opposed to actually and finally feeling it. God had a totally different plan for me than the one I was on. He saw greater things in me than I could have ever imagined. I had been playing small for years and, honestly, I think He felt it was time to yank me out of it and to create the life I really signed up for. Those walls were thick and heavy and it was quite the journey to remove them to finally see my light within.

I knew that God was up-leveling my life because I wasn't getting to where I needed to be. I had to experience my own dark night of the soul.

Ann Webb said it so eloquently: *When it's time to up-level your life, be prepared for what has been called 'the dark night of the soul.*

Your friends and family don't understand what you're going through unless they have experienced their own *dark night.*

- Whatever compassion is offered can't even begin to reach the depth of your despair.
- The path you're following has become dry as dust and clearly isn't working anymore.
- You start wondering that maybe God isn't real after all and transformation can *never* be worth this!
- You question your worthiness and your words.
- You feel completely alone and betrayed.
- Agonizing emotions convince you that you are not going to survive the hopeless state of being, and that you might die. And if you did—well, that would be perfectly ok.
- It's more than sadness, depression or anxiety.
- It's called the *dark night of the soul* because you wonder *How do I make it through the night?*
- You cry everyday.

And yet...

- You find out that every wise and enlightened person has gone through it.
- It's inescapable, and actually desirable because it's the trans-forming touch of the Spirit.

- You learn that the endurance of darkness is preparation for greater light.
- You learn that you're strong, and that the spiritual benefits of embracing it might be worth the grueling pain.
- You go to bed thinking you know something and wake up saying, *I don't know anything!*
- Your ego gives way to spirit and that's beautiful (a bad day for the ego is a good day for the soul).
- It's your refiner's fire—your Gethsemane

If you have made a commitment to God and yourself that you're ready to evolve and awaken—be prepared!

The *dark night of the soul* puts an end to your life as you know it, including the parts you wish would never change. But when you are serious to up-leveling spiritually, God will crush your ego and my advice is simply *heed*. Just surrender. It's going to be ugly and hurt like *hell*, but at the end of the day, week or even year, you are like the butterfly emerging from the chrysalis. Trust God. Thank God.

The *dark night of the soul* I experienced nearly knocked me under. But in the end, it became the beginning of a huge purging my spirit needed to get to the next level that would catapult me into the growth my spirit was crying out for so that change could finally happen.

I went to the depths of humility and I took ownership of my own actions and my own dysfunctionality that I had created in my relationship. I had to do some hard core soul searching and over-coming and letting go. I had to forgive others and forgive myself. I had to choose love instead of hatred and bitterness. I had to finally choose freedom.

It was a *looooooooooonng* road to get there, in fact it took years. I didn't know how to heal then the way I do today. After experiencing such heartache and being led on my own journey, I finally realized it didn't have to take as long to heal. I have found a deep, meaningful and more permanent healing and purpose in who I am and what I came here to do. I decided I am worth loving and I have an amazing life full of joy! This makes me a better mother, wife, sister and friend.

But my story doesn't stop there. Even after I remarried and had already found so much healing, I had several experiences that yet again knocked me over the head and shook my foundation to the very core, including another *dark night of the soul* experience. It wiped me out.

What I knew and believed in wasn't truth and I saw betrayal at the deepest level. I went through a painful experience as one lie after another unfolded about what I had believed in for the previous 20 years of my life and even into my childhood. It was devastating and painful and overwhelming to the point that my body shut down. I literally laid in bed one day where I couldn't even move my head or hands to drink a cup of water. I couldn't eat or even make sense of my thoughts. My heart was once again shattered and broken and I felt lost. I felt anguish. Anger welled up inside of me as I tried to process all that I was experiencing and all the raw emotion that felt so overwhelming and all consuming. Again, pain took my breath away.

But this time, because I had tools I didn't have before, the healing took place at a deeper level and in a more efficient and effective way. I had insight. I had experience. I had growth, and I had powerful knowledge that helped to create healing at an accelerated level without having to relive the drama or the trauma. Rather than years, this time it only took weeks to overcome and it was powerful. Instead of resisting, I went in full force and walked through it and overcame while God showed me the miracles of healing that could really take place within me. I healed energetically on a deep spiritual level and had knowledge that Christ's healing power could heal me in ways I had never before experienced. It was a whole new dimension of healing than ever before. I had to draw from a well deep within to let go of the pain and emotions that came about from the consequences of other's choices. The only way it could happen efficiently and permanently was through the healing light of Christ. It was like He took an eraser and erased the heartache and pain, cleansed my spirit and soul and the energy around me. Today, I see the same power being used in the lives of my clients and I cannot imagine a more fulfilling place to be than watching people's lives transform through the love and light of Christ that I myself experienced.

God led me on a journey to find myself, and through serving others, and really embracing Christ as my older brother, I found healing within. I'm at a place in life where I know my purpose and I know what I came here to do. Every morning I wake up excited about what I get to do that day. There is a peace that surpasses all understanding and a level of trust within me I never knew existed.

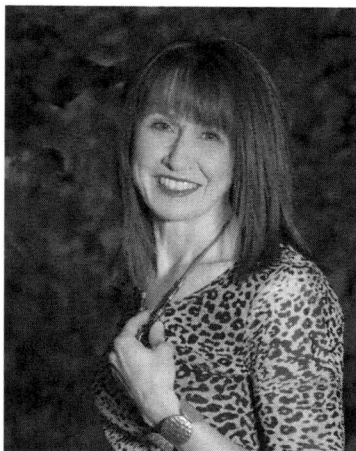

JENNIFER JONES SMITH

*Jennifer Jones Smith is a best-selling author, inspiring speaker, certified SimplyHealed®
practitioner, certified Eternal Warriors mentor and marriage consultant. She has a Professional Child Care Degree from BYU/Idaho and owned Family Circle Daycare for
20 years. Jennifer has been a coach for Hope Haven Events marriage mentoring and for
3 Key Elements Elite program.*

*As a gifted healer and mentor she works with clients to remove the self-sabotaging blocks
that keep them stuck from achieving the success they desire in their lives. Her clients
are from the continental US as well as Europe and Alaska. Visit myheartfelthealing.
com or bethetrueu.com*

I used to think of healing as the process of becoming well from
a physical ailment. I knew there was such a thing as spiritual
healing through the atonement of Christ by repentance to
cleanse one from sins. As I learned about energy healing and
became a practitioner myself, healing took on a new and powerful meaning.

Several years before I learned about energy healing I was involved in a wellness company. Many of the products they manufactured used magnetic technology to mimic earth's healing energy and to create a "wellness home" environment. Muscle testing, or applied kinesiology, was used to demonstrate the positive energy and health benefits of several of their products. Testing someone's energy to look for weakness in their energy became second nature to me, so when I attended my SimplyHealed ® energy healing training several years later, it didn't take long for me to feel comfortable using muscle testing to shift out negative trapped emotions and subconscious programming.

I chose the first modality I was trained in because I was on an email list of an entrepreneur who shared how she and her husband were having some relationship difficulties. They had an energy healing session with Carolyn Cooper, the founder of SimplyHealed®. Not only did it help their relationship, but it influenced their children in a positive way as well. When we shift our energy and vibration to a higher more positive place, it can't help but affect those around us.

I had been looking for something to expand my natural intuition and discernment and a way to create a new business venture. I felt with my background in wellness and muscle testing, I could learn energy healing and would enjoy helping others with this new skill. I quickly signed up for and completed the online basics course, and three weeks later I was in St. George, Utah, for my official hands-on training.

At my initial four-day intense training, I felt that I was on a different planet. The powerful positive energy, the shifting of negative trapped emotions, and the release of many false beliefs for me and the other students felt overwhelmingly good. How does "overwhelming" feel good? We usually think of feeling overwhelmed in a negative way. After being immersed in the healing energy of the training for several days, it was difficult to want to return to real life. However, I was taking new skills, gifts and a fresh perspective on life home with me.

Energy healing has been a blessing to me, my family and my clients. As mentioned before, I used to think of healing as mostly from injury, sickness or disease. I received a blessing in which I was told I would have the faith to be healed and to heal, and that along with that faith and my husband's priesthood, my family would be healed. I had heard many stories of pioneers and even church members being healed through priesthood power from ailments or injuries. I assumed this blessing was referring to similar things.

I have since come to realize that my inspiration to be trained in energy work was part of the manifestation of this blessing I'd received over 30 years ago. I've learned techniques to facilitate healing in my family, myself and others but more in the realm of emotional and spiritual healing which affects our physical health as well—as they are all linked together.

The adversary gives us such intense opposition. Sometimes we are pained with guilt when Satan entices us through negative thoughts and feelings to act against our values. These choices can impact our lives from mild to severe consequences. Anytime we act against who we truly are meant to be, we are in conflict with our divine self which causes emotional and often physical pain.

Other times, life presents challenges where we may feel anger, frustration, anxiety, guilt, shame, embarrassment, jealousy, envy, sadness, etc. If these emotions don't move through us or process completely, they become stuck causing low negative vibrations in the body that also show up as mental anguish and possibly physical problems. Whether our struggles and pain in life are caused by our own poor choices or just the normal opposition in life that we all face, we are all in need of spiritual and emotional healing throughout our lives.

A skilled energy healing practitioner can move trapped emotions and change subconscious false beliefs and programming quickly and easily. This gets a client into a higher more positive energy and vibration. However, as a certified mentor, I also give my clients tools that will allow them to dramatically reduce future emotional issues and even heal themselves through Christ by shifting their energy to a higher plane.

I've had many wonderful experiences of helping family and clients heal from past traumas and anxieties. However, I will share an interesting story about energy work with my birth mom. As a young junior in high school, she was taken advantage of, and that's how I came to be. I can't imagine how it must have felt for her and her parents to give up one of their own, but through their decision I had an amazing father, mother and brother who loved me immensely and treated me as their little princess.

In energy work we do "dedications," which is energy work for someone who isn't physically in our presence. We simply ask their spirit if it's alright to work on them. When we get a feeling of "yes," then we proceed with energy work and send it to them like sending a prayer to heaven. Their spirit chooses whether or not to accept it.

As a new practitioner, I remember checking on my birth mom although I had never been with her since my birth. Her energy felt to me as if she was grounded, confident and was fairly calm and happy. A year or so later I did some more energy work on her. Among other things, I found her heart chakra energy to be weak. The heart chakra has to do with love of self and others and forgiveness. Her energy didn't feel as confident and happy as it had previously, and I wondered if something was wrong in her life.

When I was 48 years old I decided to actively find her as the state of Washington opened up the birth records. I was able to get a copy of my original birth certificate. Upon finding her information, I sent a letter to her. I watched for a letter for a few weeks. However, she finally responded with a phone call. When I saw her name on the caller ID, I was excited and nervous at the same time.

We talked for several hours, and I found out her father had passed away and that she had also divorced her husband of 42 years who had been having an affair. These two events happened before the second time I had dedicated energy work to her. No wonder there was such a shift in her energy between the first and second time I had checked on her! You can imagine her feeling broken-hearted at the loss of her father and the end of her marriage. What a humbling experience to realize I connected with her on a spiritual and energetic level even though I had been disconnected from her since my birth!

Recently, I was privileged to reunite with my birth mother as she visited my home, and I later meet my two half-brothers when I visited her home. It was a pleasant, welcomed and healing reunion from both sides.

There is a weakness that energy healing work is helping me to diminish—a tendency to judge others. I actually developed this weakness later in life because I was nonjudgmental in my earlier years. As I've gotten older, and probably more critical of myself, I've become more judgmental and critical of others. Once I get to know someone, that perception diminishes dramatically.

Not judging others unrighteously is an important component of loving others with Christ-like charity. As we learn to use the atonement in our lives and not judge ourselves harshly, we can more easily accept others and have a greater power and capacity to love them.

What I LOVE about energy work is how it teaches me that no matter our weaknesses, Christ loves us all the same and wants to give us the opportunity to heal through him. I've worked on some clients who I may have criticized for their mistakes, had they been strangers in passing. However, I've been blessed to feel charity towards them, see their own pain and suffering for what it is, and have a love and compassion towards them, and a sincere gratitude for the opportunity to facilitate some healing for them through Christ.

I remember an energy healing session with a young father who dealt with pornography addiction. He had struggled for years to rid himself of this bondage. This was a vice that amongst other serious sins such as adultery or fornication, I have never been challenged with. As I look at it from a point of compassion, I realized that we all have our own wickedness to overcome, and although it appears that there are varying degrees of the severity of sins, Christ's atonement covers all levels of sin.

I am reminded of David whom we learn about in the Old Testament. This David killed the giant Goliath and was loved and revered by his people. Later in life he became one of the greatest kings in the history of Israel. He united the tribes into one nation, secured possession of the land that had been promised to his people, and set up a government based on God's law. However, the last 20 years of his life were marred by the sinful decisions he made, and according to President Marion G. Romney: "David,...though highly favored of the Lord (he was, in fact, referred to as a man after God's own heart), yielded to temptation. His unchastity led to murder, and as a consequence, he lost his families and his exaltation" (*Ensign*, may 1979, 42).

As I work with sons and daughters of God in my energy healing practice, I realize that none of us are immune from the temptations of the adversary. We must be constant and diligent in keeping the covenants we have made to keep from being bound by the chains of Satan.

This man with the pornography addiction had a tender, injured soul. I could feel the sincerity in his willingness to change and also the struggle. As we proceeded through the energy healing session, he had low self-worth, shame and guilt and struggled to love and accept himself. He also had a hard time feeling accepted, loved and valued by others. As a priesthood leader in his home, this addiction was keeping him from being the strength and anchor of righteousness that his family needed.

I was grateful to see how sensitive he was to releasing the negative energy around his struggle. Although he shed many tears and was able to release numerous trapped emotions, I'm sure he had more work to do in becoming worthy of the blessings our Father in Heaven has for him. Is this not how the atonement works for all of us? We are in a constant battle between good and evil and learning how to make ourselves more worthy of the blessings our Heavenly Father would like to bestow on us not only in the eternities, but even in our current earthly existence.

No matter our religious upbringing or beliefs, the Savior's atoning sacrifice is there for all who desire to embrace its cleansing power, and give us all hope. I am not the one to judge others and am grateful that is Christ's job. My job is to learn to love without reservation.

Christ is the healer! I'm a practitioner and simply facilitate the movement of the energy to allow Christ to heal others in His own way. I'm hoping that, at least in small increments, I am becoming purified and more like Him in unconditionally loving and serving those around me.

THE

Healer's
Call

BOOK ONE